Responsible Citizens

Responsible Citizens

Individuals, Health and Policy under Neoliberalism

B. J. Brown and Sally Baker

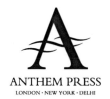

ANTHEM PRESS
LONDON · NEW YORK · DELHI

Anthem Press
An imprint of Wimbledon Publishing Company
www.anthempress.com

This edition first published in UK and USA 2012
by ANTHEM PRESS
75-76 Blackfriars Road, London SE1 8HA, UK
or PO Box 9779, London SW19 7ZG, UK
and
244 Madison Ave. #116, New York, NY 10016, USA

British Library Cataloguing-in-Publication Data
A catalogue record for this book is available from the British Library.

Library of Congress Cataloging-in-Publication Data
Brown, B. J. (Brian J.)
Responsible citizens : individuals, health, and policy under
neoliberalism / B.J. Brown and Sally Baker.
p. cm.
Includes bibliographical references and index.
ISBN 978-0-85728-458-7 (hardback : alk. paper)
1. Medical policy–Wales. 2. Health planning–Wales. I. Baker,
Sally. II. Title.
RA395.W3B76 2012
362.109429–dc23
2012005870

ISBN-13: 978 0 85728 458 7 (Hbk)
ISBN-10: 0 85728 458 4 (Hbk)

This title is also available as an eBook.

For Xylia, an inspiration, and Pete

CONTENTS

ACKNOWLEDGEMENTS

We would like to thank the numerous friends and colleagues who have spent so much time sharing their thoughts and anecdotes with us regarding the sometimes very strange direction that health and social policy has taken over recent years. We are particularly grateful to John Bailey, Graham Day, Howard Davis, Paul Evans, Martina Feilzer, Hefin Gwilym, Ian Rees Jones, Ann Krayer, Ann McLaren, Catherine Robinson, Yvonne Tommis and Fiona Zinovieff for their conversations and observations. Also, we give thanks to Marta Eichsteller, whose incredulity at what she sometimes witnesses always entertains us. Most importantly, we thank the many people who in their capacity as patients or staff – or sometimes both – of the health and social care services spoke to us in confidence regarding the customs and practices of this particular field of human endeavour, and helped to provide insight into the way in which the services worked.

PREFACE

Our interest in this subject was stimulated by the contradictions that we witnessed at a personal and local level. Perhaps the most unlikely places for neoliberal discourses to penetrate are rural communities and contradictions in policies based on neoliberal notions of individual responsibility became particularly acute when we looked through the lens of rural north Wales. The results were frequently so absurd as to be laughable, but we stopped laughing when a campaign to build a sizeable prison on the banks of the Menai Strait began in earnest, with near universal support from local politicians and the welfare services. Neoliberal penality had most certainly arrived in the UK and had taken root in the fertile soil of north Wales.

This volume draws on local, national and international sources. We finished writing this book in 2011, at a time when the UK Conservative–Liberal Democrat coalition government applied the stringent financial discipline that they promised and began to implement their programme of legislation. The pace of change is so rapid that by the time this book is published, some of the sanctions and policies that we discuss here will no longer exist. Yet the overall trend continues in the same direction – a relentlessly individualistic discourse of personal responsibility, combined with escalating levels of criminal sanction. One of us is based in north Wales and the other has close connections with the region – therefore we have selected a number of examples from Wales to illustrate the points that we make and also to show how the processes we describe are inflected and enacted differently in different areas and political cultures. As a result of devolved powers the debate is taking on a different form in Wales, although discourses of responsibility are very much in evidence from politicians and policymakers in the Welsh government. At present, the Welsh government is determined to follow a rather different path to the Westminster coalition and has a very much more positive orientation toward public services than the Westminster administration. People in Wales are being urged to exercise responsibility in order to refrain from drawing too heavily on the public services, so that provision for all will remain affordable in the face of demographic and socioeconomic changes. The coming years will be interesting, as the UK coalition and the Welsh government follow two very different paths regarding health and social policy, both using discourses of individual responsibility, to achieve very different outcomes.

Chapter One

INTRODUCTION

Setting the Scene

The individual has never been more important. In politics, education, the workplace, health and social care, leisure and almost every other sphere of public and private life the individual and his or her capacities are sovereign. Yet this importance and apparent power assigned to the individual is not all that it seems. As we shall argue here, it has gone hand in hand with a subtle authoritarianism that has insinuated itself into the government of the population. In this book we will be considering the 'public sphere' as broadly conceived, but we have a particular interest in health and social care. The trend towards individualism has been identified throughout the body politic in many nations, especially in the 'developed world', yet it is perhaps most conspicuous in health and social welfare, such that a kind of 'governance through responsibility' is enjoined upon the population.

This book documents and questions the current prevalence of individualized ways of thinking and healthcare solutions in contemporary policy in Europe and North America. Physical and mental health are conceptualized as never before as being to do with the individual's thoughts and actions. Yet this is certainly not the only way to think about health and leaves us poorly equipped to conceptualize, for example, the relationship between wellbeing and poverty or the strong connections between social cohesion, social capital and health.

Why This Book? Why Now?

The striking feature of individualism in health and social care policy is that it has colonized so much of the social fabric and so many of the ways in which we attempt to take care of ourselves and one another. This process of governance has expanded by leaps and bounds and is instantiated in far more ways than were envisaged in Nikolas Rose's germinal *Governing the Soul* (1990). It pervades considerably more of the social infrastructure than the anxieties detailed by Frank Furedi in *Therapy Culture* (2003) and whilst it is not dissimilar to *The Culture of Fear* (1997) that Furedi also identifies, we will detail instead how the idealized, responsible individual is constructed. In healthcare, responsible patients are exhorted to ensure that their bodies are managed appropriately in order to merit medical intervention. For a growing range of treatments, their weight must be judged to be appropriate, they must have given up smoking, reduced their drinking, moderated their intake of fats and be taking exercise at a level believed to be optimal. In mental healthcare especially, the role of clients and their carers has recently been invested with additional responsibilities. Clients are responsible for maintaining themselves on medication regimes which are often onerous in terms of side effects, carers are apt to be left to manage crises with minimal support and expressions of disorientation or ill temper may be met with criminal sanction. Those on benefits for incapacity or invalidity are subject to inspection and review to ensure that they meet the increasingly stringent criteria in order to receive money. In the UK they are likely to be harangued into readying themselves for employment by means of cognitive behavioural therapy (Z. Williams 2009). Individual solutions based in psychotherapy are increasingly promoted as remedies for sociopolitical disturbances and collective experiences of conflict such as terrorism.

Individualism pervades the realm of public and policy discourse, especially where health and social care are concerned. Clients who may be at their most abject and vulnerable are urged to take responsibility for themselves rather than further burden the health and social care services. In many healthcare organizations, prosecutions are mounted against clients who have lost their temper or who act inappropriately as a result of their disorientation, under the guise of 'making them take responsibility for their actions'. Citizens on the street are likely to have responsibility thrust upon them through mechanisms such as electronic surveillance and the burgeoning new cohorts of community enforcement officers, local authority officials with powers to issue fixed penalty notices and private security guards, as well as the police themselves.

This book therefore aims to explore the topography of responsibility in the early twentieth century. We undertake this task a few months into a new period in British politics, with the book going to press approximately a year after the formation of a Conservative–Liberal Democrat coalition government, following upon the heels of an unbroken 13-year New Labour regime. Meanwhile, parts of the UK such as Wales and Scotland are securing for themselves increasing financial and legislative autonomy. We will be commenting on what all this means for the formulation and exercise of responsibility. Prime minister David Cameron has regularly promoted what he calls the 'Big Society', a notion which is often hard to define but seems to involve volunteering, civic engagement and enhancement of the social fabric. He is quoted as saying, 'I just profoundly believe that in life we have obligations beyond paying taxes and obeying the law. The Big Society is about trying to create a culture where people ask "What more can I do?"' (Winnett 2011, 12). Responsible citizens are proactive paragons of civic engagement, enhancing the social fabric and selflessly crafting themselves, their families and their neighbourhoods to achieve greater economic independence, social capital and wellbeing. The responsibility agenda has therefore been continued and enhanced with the change of government as further exhortations are added to the menu of duties incumbent on the responsible citizen.

Structure of the Book

Our exploration of individualism and responsibility falls into a further eight chapters. Chapter Two lays out the conceptual tools that we will use. Definitions of individualism and neoliberalism are attempted and their relevance to contemporary political life in Europe and North America are established. We will expound the view proposed by Michel Foucault and popularized by Nikolas Rose that there are specific 'technologies of the self' at work to make up the modern individual, complete with the sense of 'choice' and 'self-determination' that is at the heart of neoliberal politics (Foucault 1980, 1985; Martin, Gutman et al. 1988; Rose 1990). Most discussions of neoliberalism have focused on the economic and political domain, with emphasis on the importance of free trade and the deregulation of markets in favour of corporate interests. Yet equally interesting are the implications for the citizen in terms of what is expected of them under such regimes and more interestingly citizens' images of themselves, as the anchors of state-stabilized institutions are gradually released. The concept of the person as someone who can be self-reliant, flexible and who can cope with the instabilities of the market by continually investing themselves with skills, abilities and preventative measures is one which has a specific genealogy. We shall explore this in Chapter Two in readiness for more extensive treatments later.

In Chapter Three, we explore some of the implications of this new age of responsibility in healthcare. Whilst the state has undertaken a withdrawal from many of the postwar consensus technologies for ensuring the health of its citizenry, this has been supplanted by a growth in discourse which places the responsibility for welfare squarely in the hands of citizens themselves. This has operated not so much through coercion but through exhorting citizens to undertake a variety of personal disciplines to manage themselves, arranging their bodies, minds and lives around the expert advice dispensed by public health bodies and government agencies. Especially for those citizens deemed to be vulnerable or 'socially excluded', notions of choice and responsibility are often accompanied by legislative frameworks through which their conduct can be regulated or normalized, and it is frequently supposed that a person's vulnerabilities arise as a result of poor personal decisions or bad habits. It is these that are often the focus of epidemiological investigation and government concern in the contemporary era.

Chapter Four delves deeper into the processes of responsibilization in healthcare, where patients and clients are being seen increasingly as rational consumers of healthcare services who are also charged with managing themselves as a potential source of risk. The risks we face are increasingly seen as personally embodied and susceptible to our participation in screening programmes, despite limited epidemiological evidence of their effectiveness. The subjective space inside the patient's or consumer's head is carved out as a realm for intervention and as a driver of the healthcare enterprise itself. Within this kind of regime, individual cognitive capacity is theorized as a key factor in wellbeing, compliance with expert advice and responsibility itself. The reach of responsibilization extends also to individuals who might, in earlier times, have been looked after entirely by statutory services, but are now being encouraged into a new brand of entrepreneurship as contemporary welfare regimes 'empower' them to organize and pay for their own care services.

In Chapter Five we will explore the notion of responsibility as it is manifested in mental healthcare. Frequently we have found that distressed people are urged to take responsibility, even when they are in hospital involuntarily. This highlights with particular acuity some of the tensions within the concept of responsibility. On the one hand, the individual is not responsible, which is why they were hospitalized, yet on the other they have responsibility thrust upon them. This is also to be seen in cases where people with mental health problems find their way into the criminal justice system, such that their disorientation, distress or disability is met with criminal sanction. Increasingly, therapeutic regimes in mental healthcare are impressing on clients that it is their responsibility to want to get better and their responsibility to do so under their own steam. The discourse of self-determination has grown strong in mental healthcare at the same time as the scale and variety of services available has, arguably, grown smaller.

Chapter Six pursues the notion of responsibility as it has been manifested in psychotherapy. A great many leading figures in twentieth-century psychotherapy have extolled the process of taking responsibility as an essential accompaniment to change. In some psychotherapeutic systems, any perceived limitation imposed by the outside world is reconfigured as the responsibility of the individual who perceives it. The individualism and preoccupation with personal wellbeing in contemporary policy is not imbibed directly from mid-twentieth-century American psychotherapy of course, but it has become part of the conceptual fabric which is readily drawn upon in the formulation of the citizen's duty to be well.

Chapter Seven explores an additional aspect of the process of responsibilization, namely what Garland (2001) has called the 'new punitiveness' and the novel ways in which recent governments have formulated and implemented a powerful range of civil and criminal sanctions which may be applied to the populace in the quest to encourage and enforce responsibility. Not only is there an impulse towards incarceration itself, but a variety of measures are activated to manage 'anti-social behaviour' in communities, residential areas and public spaces. These do not always spring from a strong democratic mandate, but in many cases it appears that the impulse to management and regulation has a momentum all of its own.

Chapter Eight delves further into what all this means for the conception of the self that is encouraged by the proliferation of responsibilities that are urged upon the individual. Whilst Giddens (1991) and Beck (1992) characterized the present era as one of reflexive individualism, it is clear that this has arisen as a result of a variety of processes with a much longer pedigree. The individualism of Protestant theology allied to the movement towards detraditionalization are believed by many authors to have prompted the present day preoccupation with crafting a lifestyle and identity. Telling one's story and confessing come to the fore in a variety of secular contexts, including the process of presenting oneself as an individual, as a kind of 'research' in academic contexts and as a source of continuity between fragmented experiences of work and transient relationships. Moreover, the individual is urged by a variety of media – self-help literature, popular advice from experts and even talk show hosts – that 'opening up' is somehow beneficial. Moreover, a good deal of popular advice is directed towards lowering expectations of material advancement and instead focusing on the inner rearrangement of values to secure 'fulfilment' or 'resilience' for the individual.

Taken together, these processes encourage the citizen to be self-fulfilling and self-developing almost as if this were a social obligation, as we argue in Chapter Nine. The obligation to self-development as part of citizenship has been underscored by David Cameron in his 2010 party conference speech. Equally, the coalition government has embraced the notion of 'nudging' people toward expert-approved, politically expedient modes of conduct, following Thaler and Sunstein's (2008) book of the same name. The responsible citizen is not one who can genuinely claim autonomy, but rather one who conducts himself or herself as directed or nudged by a variety of experts and government agencies. As Hunter (1996) presciently claimed over a decade and a half ago, this is the era of the 'pedagogical state' and our task as citizens is to manage ourselves according to this instruction. In tandem with this, there has been a withdrawal on the part of public agencies from fields which might, under the old welfarist model, have been collective, rather than individual

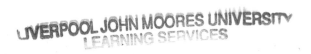

responsibilities. Rather than heal us when we become sick, health services are likely to see their role as dispensing 'healthy living' advice. In the event of tragedies in child protection or social care, subtle shifts in accountability are undertaken so that it is the clients themselves who bear the responsibility. Practices of audit, inspection and review, ostensibly to enhance accountability and value for money across a variety of public services, have gone hand in hand with a shrinkage in the range and variety of problems which public services can tackle. Accompanying this is a sense of what Hirschorn (1997) has called 'market risk', such that practitioners no longer feel confident in their own capabilities in the face of the liabilities involved in their practice.

Thus, a picture emerges of contemporary citizens who are urged to be responsible yet at the same time to rely on expert guidance, education and nudges, governed by legislative frameworks that are apt to be punitive and who are encouraged to think of themselves as vulnerable and in need of assistance. This brings the citizen into a new kind of relationship with him or herself – a relationship that is mediated by expertise or by the state itself.

Of course, the citizen is not always compliant in the face of the sheer minatory power of the state or of expert advice. Educators and policymakers are almost always disappointed by the uptake of advice, whether this be to do with eating fruit and vegetables, participating in health screening programmes, becoming volunteers, taking exercise or clearing up after their dogs. The penetration of these practices is always incomplete. Yet the significance is in the new ways that they afford of conceptualizing citizens, or of thinking about ourselves in relation to assemblages of expertise, processes of governance and society itself.

Nor should we see an authoritarian conspiracy at work every time a doctor advises a patient to give up smoking, a housing officer tries to get tenants to keep the noise down, exasperated neighbours call the police about rowdy teenagers or politicians, frustrated at the intractability of economic problems, urge us to concentrate on self-fulfilment instead. Taken separately, these are relatively banal everyday incidents. Yet collectively, across a variety of sites and a myriad of occasions, we would argue that they add up to something more. Rather than an authoritarian conspiracy, this perhaps reflects what Nikolas Rose (1999) and before him Michel Foucault (1990) would see as the 'capillary' nature of power. The practices are locally implemented and are true in a much more particular sense than if they resulted from the imposition of some wide ranging ulterior fiat. As Rose's collaborator Peter Miller describes in his work on what he calls the 'calculating self', the continual process of evaluation, economic reckoning and self-measurement peculiar to the modern age goes hand in hand with the shaping of subjectivity or forms of personhood (Miller and Rose 2008). This provides new possibilities for acting on oneself and on the actions of others.

Certainly, this process does not always work seamlessly. The 'technologies' (in Foucault's terms) with which personhood can be shaped are always to a greater or lesser degree ineffective, either through outright resistance or through their failure to gain sufficient purchase on the public imagination. The instruments for the governance of conduct and the rationalities that articulate the aims and objectives of governing may frequently encounter limits regarding what can be done (Mennicken 2008). The ideas of audit, inspection and scrutiny seem today to travel effortlessly across a vast range of territories (Power 1997). But other devices, for instance thinking through the lens of structural inequalities, seem to travel with increasing difficulty. This suggests that we still have much to find out about how the different dimensions of the responsible self travel and how this peculiarly modern form of personhood is fashioned and refashioned in historically specific assemblages. Thus we want to point to a degree of consilience between the variety of practices which seek to manage health risks, operationalize and shape desirable conduct and specify a desired mindset on the part of citizens, because as Miller and Rose (1994, 59) state, this process constitutes an 'ability to spread a particular way of understanding, judging and intervening over a wide surface of practices and issues'. Moreover, this has the potential to 'redefine the limits of vision, and create new ways of acting upon that which is brought into view.'

It is therefore our ambition in this book to look at how responsibility and citizenship are shaped and contoured around these issues. Whilst we cannot of course tell exactly how it feels at firsthand for everyone under advanced liberalism, we can certainly sketch the variety of official and popular discourses unfolding at the present time, the kinds of preferences which are being expressed for citizens' conduct, the technologies which are being put in place to make visible and shape behaviour, the forms of personhood which are called into being and the implications this has for notions of authority as we move deeper into the twenty-first century.

Chapter Two

INDIVIDUALISM, NEOLIBERALISM AND THE IMPERATIVES OF PERSONAL GOVERNANCE

In this chapter we will lay out some of the key concepts and tools that we will be using over the course of this book. Many of the core notions such as individualism, neoliberalism, citizenship and the process of responsibilization itself have already generated large and growing literatures of their own and we can merely scratch their respective surfaces. Nevertheless, it is valuable to adumbrate some of the key features as they will be informing our discussion later in the volume. Many of these ideas did not spring to life fully formed. Rather, they are the product of specific intellectual histories, as commentators, educators, policymakers and individuals themselves sought to make sense of what was happening in particular cultures at specific moments. Nevertheless, they have played important parts in contemporary social and political drama, and have often been among the principal sites, objects and instruments of responsibilization. Let us begin with the oldest concept to bear its present name, that of individualism.

Individualism

American scholars such as Bellah, Madsen et al. (1985) point to the nineteenth-century French social philosopher Alexis de Tocqueville (1805–1859) as the originator of the term 'individualism'. Tocqueville coined the term following his government-sponsored nine month visit to survey the American prison system (Triandis 1995, 20).

In Tocqueville's *Democracy in America*, the first volume of which was published in 1835, he described individualism as arising as a result of the loss of an older system where social worlds were more overtly hierarchical. The old style aristocratic chain of dependencies and responsibilities continually reinforced an individual's awareness of others and encouraged forgetfulness of self (Tocqueville [1835] 1969, 507). In Tocqueville's view, a society of equals in which individuals are expected to support themselves turns everyone's thoughts to themselves.

This encourages a withdrawal from society at large (Tocqueville [1835] 1969, 508). Thus even as he described it, Tocqueville entertained some misgivings about individualism. The focus on the self and one's immediate family group undermined the possibilities for participatory government. As he noted:

> ...I see an innumerable multitude of men, alike and equal, constantly circling around in pursuit of the petty and banal pleasures with which they glut their souls. Each of them withdrawn into himself, is almost unaware of the fate of the rest. Mankind, for him, consists in his children and his personal friends. As for the rest of his fellow citizens, they are near enough, but he does not notice them. He touches them but feels nothing. He exists in and for himself, and though he still may have a family, one can at least say that he has not got a fatherland. (Tocqueville [1835] 1969, 692)

These misgivings are echoed in the contemporary era by authors such as Bellah, Madsen et al. (1985) who draw on Tocqueville's analysis of American individualism to undergird their own concern about the growth of individualism in America. They believe that this leads to 'cancerous' and 'dangerous' effects on communities and the nation as a whole. The tendency within individualism for citizens to withdraw and isolate themselves from others is, in their view, a trend that weakens the entire society.

At the same time, there were a number of intellectual tendencies from the Enlightenment onward that saw individualism as an important value to be promoted. Kim (2009) identifies 'utilitarian individualism' that can be traced to Benjamin Franklin. This focuses primarily on individual self-improvement through material resources. This tendency, stressing the virtue of perpetual toil and self-improvement, is one to which we shall return later in this book, especially as it can be found in a good deal of contemporary social and health policy.

As Kim (2009) also notes, individualism has a strong expressive strand. This emphasizes the pursuit of individualism as a means of capturing some notional true selfhood or personal identity. Expressive individualism is represented in the American tradition by Ralph Waldo Emerson (1803–1882), Henry David Thoreau (1817–1862) and Walt Whitman (1819–1892). Here, selfhood represents a kind of quest narrative such that by regaining and recapturing selfhood a person can become who he or she sets out to be or who he or she 'really' is. In this view as Kim (2009, 567) notes, 'individualism is the key to liberating persons and ushering them into perfection'. While Emerson's views have been described as neglecting the sufferings and pain of the world (Arieli 1964), they chimed in with those of many American and European commentators at the time. Michel Chevalier (1806–1879), a French engineer, economist and contemporary of Tocqueville, had a much more positive outlook than the latter on American individualism. Chevalier was particularly inspired by individualism in relation to the revolt against authority in religion, politics and society (Arieli 1964). He therefore considered the flourishing American individualism to be a creative and liberating product of the Protestant revolution.

In celebration of the quest of individualism Capps (1993) asserts, with Emerson (1979), that the self is subject to a much loftier and higher calling than mere social conformity. An overweening concern with other people and their wants, needs and expectations may cause individuals to lose their true selves and develop a 'false self' characterized by the loneliness that will emerge instead. For thinkers in the Emersonian tradition, individualism is not the cause of an individual's loneliness or isolation, but the beginning of its amelioration. Further support for this understanding can be found in Coleman (1982) and Sennett (1980), who suggest that it is modern social organizations such as institutions and corporations, not an unchecked individualism, that drive individuals into isolation. It is soulless contemporary bureaucracies pushing individuals into becoming 'corporate actors' who are mere extensions of their companies and who must suppress their true selves and characters. In contrast, this expressive individualism is seen by Bellah, Madsen et al. (1985) as a particularly destructive force, inasmuch as it is a form of self-expression that promotes celebrating the self above all things and therefore poses a threat to society. The pursuit of self-discovery and self-realization erodes family and community relationships and encourages a weakening of the social fabric. This is another theme to which we shall return later. From our point of view, a notable consequence of the expressive individualist tradition is how it has slipped so readily into social and political thinking.

This tendency to see the individual as logically and ontologically prior to the social scene was a concern of Lukes (1973) in his landmark work *Individualism*. He describes his quarry:

According to this conception, individuals are pictured abstractly as given, with given interests, wants, purposes, needs, etc.; while society and the state are pictured as sets of actual or possible social arrangements which respond more or less adequately to those individuals' requirements. Social and political rules and institutions are, on this view, regarded collectively as an artifice, a modifiable instrument, a means of fulfilling independently given individual objectives; the means and the end are distinct. The crucial point about this conception is that the relevant features of individuals determining the ends which social arrangements are held...to fulfil, whether these features are called instincts, faculties, needs, desires, rights, etc., are assumed as given, independently of a social context. (Lukes 1973, 73)

Following the aspirations described by the philosophers and poets of the nineteenth century, such as Emerson, Thoreau and Whitman, a number of commentators on the idea of individualism in the twentieth and twenty-first centuries have emphasized how this search for the self is no longer the preserve of a few intellectuals and visionaries, but has become a mass project involving substantial sections of the population. For Giddens (1991) the pursuit of self-identity is a central project of contemporary society. Giddens (1991, 215) asserts that:

> Self-identity today is a reflexive achievement. The narrative of self-identity has to be shaped, altered and reflexively sustained in relation to changing circumstances of social life, on a local and global scale.

This self-aware, self-referential creation of an identity is not, for Giddens, an entirely individualized process. Drawing on Wittgenstein, he suggests that it is through being part of a linguistic community and through intersubjectivity that we develop the capacity for subjectivity itself (Giddens 1991, 51). In spite of this, he sees the process of acquiring autonomy as involving the transcendence of interdependence and reciprocity. He distinguishes between what he calls an 'externally referential' system of norms and morals characterizing pre-modern society and modernity being characterized by a set of 'internally referential' values chosen by the individual. Hence, his idea of a 'pure relationship' – a sign of high modernity – is characterized by trust that 'by definition' is not based on kinship, social duty or traditional obligation (Giddens 1991, 6). Giddens approvingly points to the notion that reflexivity '...should produce...insightful self-knowledge and help reduce dependence in close relationships' (1991, 93). Whilst Giddens is perhaps one of its great enthusiasts, the notion of the individual making progress towards autonomy and a reduced dependence on others, developing an autonomous and unitary self, is reinforced in a good deal of liberal social theory in which the individual is perceived to face endless, fluid choices based on 'lifestyle', rather than a moral framework derived from values associated with family, religion or tradition (Giddens 1991).

In this view, the person is progressively disembedded from earlier forms of social relations of solidarity and from collective and community ties and identities (Bauman 2000; Beck 1992; Giddens 1991). As a result of this, the individual is forced to take on the responsibility of negotiating a path through the dilemmas of modern life and assemble a self-identity and biography that reflects a life of one's own choosing (Beck 1992; Beck and Beck-Gernsheim 2002; Giddens 1991). Inasmuch as this is a conscious self-aware process, the self is a 'reflexive project'; the individual decides between multiple, often conflicting, forms of information and knowledge and a field of 'choices' – increasingly enshrined in social policy – in deciding how to live (Giddens 1991; Rose 1999).

The degree of self-reflexivity involved in the construction of identities has been enhanced through the undermining of traditional forms of expertise and the development of consumer culture. Individuals are presented with ever more diverse forms of knowledge, expertise and authority from which to choose. Choice is a central precept in patients' treatment seeking within the NHS, but it also extends to a growing variety of treatment and healing options in the complementary and alternative medicine sector and the varieties of spiritual comfort available. Thus there are a variety of competing sources of knowledge and authority when it comes to understanding one's body, one's symptoms or one's place in the universe. Given this bewildering abundance of choices the processes of individualization 'not only permit, but they also demand an active contribution by individuals' (Beck and Beck-Gernsheim 2002, 4).

In connection with these processes in the health, wellbeing and social care fields, a whole variety of consumption, lifestyle and leisure activities are presented as matters in which individuals can make choices and are especially important in this process of self-production in the face of the declining value attached to the traditional anchors for identity, such as occupation, region or religious affiliation (Giddens 1991; Rose 1990).

In line with the expressive individualism discussed earlier, the individual's job is to assemble a biography for themselves. As Beck and Beck-Gernsheim (2002, 3) note, in a world that is rapidly changing, the 'do-it-yourself' biography is always a 'risk biography', indeed a 'tightrope biography'. The corollary of self-responsibility is that the causes of failure are seen as being located within the individual. Thus social and political issues can be reformulated as psychological ones. Bauman describes the state of these new citizens:

> If they fall ill, it is because they were not resolute or industrious in following a health regime. If they stay unemployed, it is because they failed to learn the skills of winning an interview or because they did not try hard enough. (Bauman 2002, xvi)

It is within this context that strategies of governance may become particularly sharply focused to manage those individuals who are believed not to be meeting their obligations as active and self-responsible citizens in ensuring their own wellbeing (Rose 1999). Those who appear not to be employed, who seem to be problematic as tenants or patients or whose engagement with schemes to make them better parents is patchy, may be subject to special scrutiny and intensive intervention.

Curiously, despite the degree of scrutiny and intervention aimed at the problematic individual, a good deal of this intervention is aimed at enjoining the individual to manage their personal condition. A television programme in the UK at the time of writing entitled *The Fairy Jobmother* (Channel 4 2010), detailed an intervention in which an unemployed couple in Middlesborough were advised by 'employment expert' Hayley Taylor. By concealing scars and coaching them on matters such as posture, how they walked, handshake and eye contact, she succeeded in getting one member of the couple a job. Whilst this focus on individual characteristics, bodily hexis and employability was staged for the television programme, it is redolent of a much broader process of governmentally sanctioned intervention aimed at making people more 'responsible' and self-reliant. Advice of a similar nature can be regularly found in the pages of local papers alongside job adverts. In 'JobsWales', a weekly feature of the *Daily Post* on 4 November 2010, the headline of the lead article informed readers that 'Voice Training is Sound Advice for Career Success', the article explaining how valuable 'voice training' is in order to improve one's career prospects. The advice was dispensed by 'executive presence coach' Elizabeth Kuhnke, 'author of the best-selling book *Body Language for Dummies*'. North Wales has for many years experienced a high level of unemployment and at the time that this feature was published the vast majority of jobs advertised in the region were casual or part-time poorly paid jobs often with employment agencies, such as for care assistants or cleaners. Interestingly, an increasingly high proportion of the few full-time or more highly paid positions are those that involve 'preparing' people in receipt of benefits for work. The edition of the *Daily Post* promoting the benefits of voice training also advertised a position for a 'fit for work service manager' 'to give people in early stages of sickness absence support to return to work earlier than they otherwise would'.

Anyone familiar with north Wales will know that the ability to communicate in Welsh would be very much more useful in securing employment in the region than 'voice training' or the sort of advice dispensed by the Fairy Jobmother. Yet such features in the jobs section of the local papers in north Wales are now common, much of the advice clearly being aimed at women. These articles are often accompanied by a photograph of a stereotypical 'career woman' or an older woman looking curiously reminiscent of a 1980s 'power dresser'. In this way, the programme exemplifies a trend in the contemporary labour market which has been termed 'aesthetic labour', whereby potential employees are enjoined to adopt particular 'embodied capacities and attributes' (Warhurst and Nickson 2001, 13) that enable employees to 'look good and sound right' for the job (2001, 2).

In Dean's terms, such interventions and advice 'illustrate how government is crucially concerned to modify a certain space marked out by entities such as…the personality, character, capacities, levels of self-esteem and motivation the individual possesses' (Dean 1999, 12). In tandem with this, Dean notes how governments and employers are encouraging a sense of independence from social movements too. Mass participation in trade union movements, political parties or campaigns and protests advocating social and economic reform is subtly and sometimes not so subtly discouraged. This is reinforced in neoliberal critiques of the welfare state and the alleged dependency that it fosters, that discloses 'a conception of freedom that moves away from the emancipatory aspirations of social movements towards the virtuous, disciplined, and responsible autonomy of the citizenry' (Dean 1999, 151).

Dean neatly anticipated the flavour of much twenty-first century policy when he said that one of the characteristics of advanced liberal governance is that 'it cedes responsibility to paternalism for those who, for whatever reason, cannot or do not exercise responsible choices' (Dean 1999, 207). There is an expectation, or even a financially sanctioned obligation, upon individuals to take up the proffered assistance. In welfare reforms in the UK, disabled people were to be penalized through reduction in benefits if they failed to 'continuously engage' in some kind of work based activity (Department for Work and Pensions 2006).

The rationales of governance established by the 1997–2010 UK New Labour government and continued by the Conservative–Liberal Democrat coalition, rest upon a notion of agency, autonomy and self-responsibility as being somehow inherent requirements of 'good' citizenship. The idea of responsibility takes on an ethical dimension in that it valorizes certain kinds of desirable conduct. It foregrounds a focus on subjects as reflexive, rational consumers and an increasing moral emphasis on citizens as duty-owing members of communities. Yet these communities are not seen as organic forms of social solidarity but as places where members' relations with each other are mediated by the state. Anti-Social Behaviour Orders (ASBOs), bans on drinking and smoking in public and semi-public spaces, vetting by the Independent Safeguarding Authority (ISA), and legislation governing the performance of live music are only a few of the means by which the social relationships and activities which might once have arisen spontaneously are now mediated by the state. In housing too the role of local authorities and housing associations in the UK is increasingly redefined in terms of the governance of conduct – not merely in terms of whether one pays one's rent or annoys one's neighbours but in terms of whether prospective tenants make a desirable addition to the 'community', which has become the location and mechanism of social housing governance (Rose 2001; Flint 2003). 'At no time since the advent of social housing has more effort been put into dividing the anti-social from those who conform to the norm' (Cowan and Marsh 2005, 40–1). We return to explore this in more detail later in this volume.

Across a range of locations and forms of private and public life the levers of government are seen by policymakers as means of securing a particular kind of desirable conduct:

> Increasingly the new politics is about moderating behaviour and re-establishing the social virtues of self-discipline coupled with an awareness of the needs of others…the new politics centre on reinforcing what is good and acceptable behaviour. (Field 2003, 1)

As a consequence, those who fail to satisfy the conditions prescribed by policymakers can be characterized as morally irresponsible, personally culpable for their failure to take responsibility for their conduct, and as such undeserving of the benefits and opportunities afforded the 'law abiding citizen'.

Neoliberalism

In line with the spirit of neoliberalism, personal conduct and even private thoughts are market commodities. Being able to demonstrate that one has conducted oneself responsibly and adopted an approved mindset can be exchanged for other kinds of goods and services via state agencies. Conduct is in a sense capitalized because it has this kind of exchange value. This aligns with the sociopolitical philosophy of neoliberalism, such that market ideology is extended beyond the production of goods and services to infuse an increasing range of social interactions as if they were market transactions (Harvey 2003). As well as drawing upon a network of discursive practices to promote the mobility of capital, neoliberalism encourages a reconceptualization of society and social life that theoretically and frequently in practice moves closer and closer to an idealized image of a free market based on an 'individualist micro-economic model' (Bourdieu 1998, 9).

This image of deregulation and market freedom has been central to the appeal of neoliberalism to policymakers, investors and global entrepreneurs over the last two decades. In 1990, John Williamson coined the term 'Washington Consensus' to describe a suite of 'policy measures about whose proper deployment Washington can muster a reasonable degree of consensus' (Williamson 1990, 10). This term originally appealed to scholars seeking to make sense of the topography of power which seemed to underlie the 1980s global 'structural adjustments' (Peet 2007). Peck and Tickell (2002) describe this 'roll back neoliberalism' (after the well-used phrase 'rolling back the state') in order to describe the situation in which 'state power was mobilized behind marketization and deregulation projects, aimed particularly at the central institutions of the Keynesian-welfarist settlement' (Peck and Tickell 2002, 388).

Especially in the US, but also in many other 'Western' economies, the discourse of neoliberalism has proved to be particularly attractive as a compelling narrative that mandates shifts from governmental responsibility to individual responsibility, from injunction to expert advice, and from centralized government to quasi-governmental agencies and media, including television, as sources of information, evaluation and reproach (Shugart 2010, 112). Proponents of neoliberalism describe welfare provision as restricting citizens by fostering dependency and contrast this with the benefits of choice – especially consumer choice – and individual fulfilment (Sender 2006, 135). So pervasive has this new planetary vulgate become that even influential figures within sociology such as Anthony Giddens (2000) have accepted that welfare creates dependency and argue instead for a concept of positive welfare 'to which individuals themselves and other agencies besides government contribute', as well as arguing that welfare 'is not in essence an economic concept but a psychic one' (Giddens 2000, 117). He proposes a 'social investment state' rather than a welfare state, whose purpose is to invest in human capital with the provision that counselling is apt to be more effective than direct economic support.

Welfare needs are reconfigured as being part of the psychic sphere rather than the economic one and concerned with the acceptance of reduced prosperity rather than its amelioration through welfare benefits, state intervention to sustain employment or even any convincing vision for investment or economic growth. Within neoliberal economic discourse 'workforce flexibility' is presented as an inevitable and desirable goal (Martin 1994). The important task for the individual under neoliberal ideology is a process of reconfiguring the self such that emotions – particularly those that might disrupt productivity or consumption, for example grief, anger or misery – are construed as something to be self-managed, privatized and constrained. 'In this way, the goals and needs of the state are positioned as congruent with those of the individual, both of which would be organized in accordance with the logic of the market' (Cox, Long et al. 2008, 476). The notion of neoliberalism is, in an important sense, a psychological one involving a reconfiguration not only of economies, world trade arrangements and welfare systems, but of attitudes, values, projects of the self and identities too. It is in this way that neoliberalism links with the other key notion central to this book, that of responsibility or 'responsibilization'.

Neoliberalism is clearly not a cut-and-dried matter. Indeed, looking at the debates which have followed the publication of volumes such as David

Harvey's *The Enigma of Capital* (2010) or Raymond Plant's *The Neo-Liberal State* (2009) it is clear that there is little consensus concerning the drivers of political economy in the contemporary world. The key enthusiasts for the free economy and the 'liberalized markets' model of governance have long gone from the political scene. This was originally associated with politicians such as Ronald Reagan, Margaret Thatcher and General Pinochet and with economists such as Milton Friedman and Friedrich Hayek. The ethos of the 'small state' is at odds with the way that around a third to a half of the economic activity in many developed economies is accounted for by state spending (Kenny 2011) and the boundaries between state and private economic activities are blurred by the increasing use of private contractors to provide public services. Monetarism ceased to be a major force in economic policy in most developed nations some 20 years ago: 'By 1992, monetarist and rational expectations theorists had lost virtually all influence over actual policy, in the United States and elsewhere' (Krugman 2004, 197). The elements of neoliberalism then need not be present all at the same time and same place. It could be argued that neoliberalism is sufficiently supple to be a social technology as well as an economic one. It is the increasingly pervasive notions of individualism, markets and marketability acting as a cultural rubric that are perhaps the key legacies of neoliberalism (Giroux 2004) and which have led to the ascendance of markets as a metaphor to guide and drive human affairs (Chomsky 2011). It is in relation to this social sense of neoliberalism that the idea of citizens being responsible gains particular purchase.

Responsibilization

The term 'responsibilization' is appearing with increasing frequency in accounts of management, social policy, health and welfare. The concept was probably first used in the social sciences by Burchell (1996) and Garland (1996). In an early deployment of the term, Grey (1997, 719) explained that it was about rendering people 'trustworthy and predictable by virtue of their beliefs and behaviours'. Key to this responsibilization is the process of giving people knowledge or information as their initiation into some sort of technical expertise. As Grey argues, it is not because this knowledge necessarily assists their working or personal lives but it is part of a Foucauldian process of rendering them docile. Responsibilization is thus aligned with governmentality, a notion originating in Foucault's writing, denoting a form of political power comprising a range of technologies, mentalities and rationalities of governing others and oneself (Foucault 1991). Governmentality involves the state 'acting on the manner in which individuals regulate their own behaviour' (Hindess 1996, 106).

Under neoliberal regimes, the process of governmentality involves both facilitating and restricting the conduct of citizens by increasing their capacity for freedom and self-government (Rose 1999; Dean 2002, 119) Responsibilization involves the state encouraging or compelling individuals to acknowledge and assume a degree of responsibility for managing their own risks (Burchell 1996, 29). This devolution of responsibility and the emphasis on self-management does not mean that the state has entirely lost interest in individuals' conduct. Responsibilization is not equivalent to anarchy nor is it entirely equivalent to self-help, although this might form a part of the process. Rather the neoliberal state legislates to establish the rules and boundaries for such self-management. In addition, the state seeks to increase the citizens' capacity for self-management because this is believed to best serve society's interests; responsibilization underscores the duty of the prudent and rational citizen to avoid becoming a burden on others (O'Malley 1996, 200; Kemshall 2002, 42).

As Clarke (2005, 451) notes, the idea of 'rights and responsibilities' came to the fore in the UK New Labour (1997–2010) administration. Citizens were explicitly formulated as being the bearers of responsibilities as well as rights. These responsibilities were often substantial and wide-ranging, but generally revolved around 'the responsibility to produce the conditions of one's own independence – ideally by becoming a "hard working" individual or family' (Clarke 2005, 451). Importantly for the present volume, Clarke notes how citizens are enjoined to exercise their freedoms responsibly, for example by not overeating or binge drinking. Members of communities must avoid anti-social conduct in the interests of ensuring harmony, inclusivity and civility. Parents are urged to be responsible for controlling and civilizing their children and ensuring that they attend school. Citizens are urged to exercise 'reasonable' and 'responsible' choices when making use of public services so as not to 'waste' taxpayers' money.

Lowenheim (2007) identifies three main modes within the process of responsibilization. The first is found when the state retracts from its traditional roles and duties. This is especially the case where health and welfare are concerned, for example where aspects are privatized or where 'partnerships' are created between the state, the community and entrepreneurs or private investors for the joint management of risk or provision of service (Garland 1996; Ilkan and Basok 2004; Zedner 2006, 87). In the UK, this process can be seen in health and social care but also increasingly in the criminal justice system. This state withdrawal aided by the logic of the market is believed to prompt private individuals and non-state bodies to be more active and assume a growing responsibility for risk management in a given sphere. Thus, within the framework created by the state and the market, citizens 'promote individual and national well-being by their responsibility and enterprise' (Rose 1999, 139).

A second theme in responsibilizing citizens says Lowenheim (2007), involves linking the 'responsible' conduct of individual citizens (as defined by the state) with their right to avail themselves of state-provided services, benefits or protections. For example, policymakers might make the right to welfare benefits conditional on the participation of unemployed citizens in various 'empowerment' and 'return to work' programmes or make access to healthcare procedures conditional upon a patient losing weight or giving up smoking (McDonald and Marston 2005).

Finally, a third theme in the policy of responsibilization is for the state to propagate risk knowledge with the aim of increasing the individual capacity for what the state deems as responsible free choice. This knowledge in turn should be employed by the citizenry to guide their individual conduct. Thus, campaigns to introduce more legible food labelling schemes so that shoppers can see at a glance whether the product is low, medium or high in fat, sugar and salt (Maryon-Davies 2009) are intended to place more risk knowledge at the disposal of the consumer. Governmental campaigns and advice on how to maintain good health can be seen as this kind responsibilization, the propagation of this sort of knowledge emphasizing the individual's 'duty to be well' (O'Malley 2004, 72–4).

Whilst advice of this kind is widely dispensed on a whole variety of issues, the scientific basis of the advice given is not always clear-cut. To take just one example in the UK, campaigns to make consumers aware of the hazards of eating more than six grams of salt are well established, yet one key meta-analysis of studies concerning advice to reduce salt intake concluded that 'Intensive interventions, unsuited to primary care or population prevention programmes, provide only small reductions in blood pressure and sodium excretion, and effects on deaths and cardiovascular events are unclear' (Hooper, Bartlett et al. 2002). Hooper, Bartlett et al. maintain that the value of such interventions lies in allowing patients with hypertension and who are already taking drugs for this to reduce their dependence on medication and control their blood pressure via diet. So the likely effectiveness of a generic campaign directed at the general population in reducing blood pressure or on morbidity and mortality is considerably less clear. Thus the role of the advice is more to do with responsibilizing the population than in the practical results that such a process may have in terms of their health. In this regard, the process of responsibilization has a particularly interesting aspect. It is not necessarily about reductions in mortality and morbidity of practical magnitude but is about instituting particular kinds of relations between the individual, the state and the 'expertise' of advisers and health educators. Accordingly, we will move on to a consideration of how notions of responsibility are formulated and enacted in current policy discourse.

Citizenship

Citizens are generally said to be at the core of policy, yet it is often a little difficult to define exactly who they are and what they do. Citizenship education has been part of the educational curriculum in England and Wales for some time, and in one form or another has found its way into educational curricula in the four home nations of the UK with the broad aim to 'increase political engagement amongst young people and encourage an inclusive framework of civic identities' (Andrews and Mycock 2007, 74).

As Bellamy (2008) notes, citizenship was once defined in terms of a particular suite of rights, as befitted membership of a political community, whose members were entitled to take part on an equal footing with others in making decisions about collective life. This kind of focus on rights was also central to Marshall's (1963) focus on citizenship as comprising civil, political and social rights. Especially in its political aspect, citizenship was concerned with some sort of participation in democratic or civic processes, especially voting. By the middle years of the twentieth century there was a strong sense of collective solidarity – in Beveridge's words, 'winning freedom from want needs courage and faith and a sense of national unity that can override the interest of any class or section' (Beveridge 1942, 173).

In earlier conceptions there was a sense that collective solidarity through commonly held rights underscored citizenship. More recently, citizenship has been seen more in terms of social and moral dimensions, which have come to supplant the role of citizens in holding the state to account. As Eckert (2011, 310) says: 'What we are witnessing is the diminishment of state accountability, particularly in terms of the social rights of citizens'. Yet at the same time, there has been a proliferation of ways in which persons are created as legal and civil subjects by the minute administrative practices and classifications of everyday life. This could be seen as a process of étatisation – or growing state dominance – over a variety of spheres, including minds and bodies (Mitchell 1999), and governmentality which in this context refers to both the art of government and the way that governments attempt to produce those kinds of citizens best suited to fulfilling the government's policies (Rose 1999; Rose and Osborne 2000; Rose and Novas 2004).

In addition to this, the boundaries of what comprises the state in relation to the citizen are growing fuzzier. As Eckert (2011) reminds us, a variety of processes such as outsourcing, subcontracting, devolving and delegating have made the precise responsibilities and duties of the state more difficult to trace at the same time as facilitating the growth of alliances and linkages of governance in capillary fashion through the body politic. Allied to this, the more diffuse nature of many contemporary governance constellations means that it is possible for governing bodies to shift responsibility from one to the other or deflect liability (Randeria 2007; Sidakis 2009). The claims which the state can make on the citizen have become 'flexibilised' (Ong 1998), whilst at the same time the possibilities of citizens making equivalent claims on their states have become less clear-cut and as Das (2004) says, more 'illegible'. Nevertheless, there are a variety of manoeuvres through which states and citizens themselves might code and constitute each other. Rights and responsibilities might wax and wane as they are continuously negotiated, instantiated, practised and claimed by everyday acts of citizenship.

Following Das (2011), perhaps it is valuable to consider citizenship and its attendant rights and responsibilities as being created through everyday state and citizen practices such as granting tenancies in social housing, administering justice, visiting the doctor, being a member of a voluntary or civic organization and so on. In particular, for the purposes of this book, we will be interested in what it means to be a healthy citizen, a responsible tenant and a proficient participant in a variety of therapeutic and wellbeing-enhancing activities, as it is these that the capillary state has been particularly active in infiltrating. The rights and responsibilities of the citizen vis-à-vis the state are not necessarily collective any longer, but are nonetheless fundamentally social: the understanding of responsibilities and rights and the perception of oneself as a responsible or rights-bearing individual, are founded through social relations, collectively with others or by comparison to others.

Citizenship was once formulated in terms of rights that were collectively held and enjoyed, often as a result of possessing the legally sanctioned capacity to vote. More recently, this has been supplemented by a greater focus in many spheres of public discourse on the responsibilities of citizenship too; responsibilities exercised through new forms of subjection in workplaces, in public and in private life.

The Policy Context

In popular journalism and policymaking circles alike, the need for responsibility to be taken is adumbrated by a great many commentators. Where employment is concerned, journalist Jenny McCartney writes of the corrosive effect of

> the work-shaped hole in the lives of countless families and individuals that have never been encouraged – economically or otherwise – to take responsibility for themselves. Why go to bed early when you have nothing to get up for? Even taking the children to school can become a chore.

The state, believing itself compassionate, has created a permanent underclass of adults reduced to the status of half-neglected, resentful children. (McCartney 2010a, 22)

Whist this is a piece of 'mere' popular journalism it includes some important arguments. The individual and their wellbeing are defined in relation to work as if this were somehow essential to human wellbeing. Long gone are the optimistic predictions of the 1970s that with increasing mechanization and computerization we would be able to look forward to a life where leisure predominated over work. Now work is central. There is also a notion that the absence of work leads to a creeping neglect of other responsibilities. If work is absent, then taking children to school will be the next item to fail.

Health especially is an area where discourses of responsibility are frequently mobilized. The need for responsibility on the part of patients is enshrined in the NHS constitution. For example:

You should recognise that you can make a significant contribution to your own, and your family's, good health and well-being, and take some personal responsibility for it. (NHS 2009, 9)

Compliance with professional advice is also mandated in the NHS constitution, which retains an expert-driven model of care in line with the reliance upon expertise noted by commentators on neoliberalism:

You should follow the course of treatment which you have agreed and talk to your clinician if you find this difficult. (NHS 2009, 9)

Behaviour in NHS facilities is subject to stipulations too, identifying the kind of deportment demanded of clients in the system.

You should treat NHS staff and patients with respect and recognise that causing a nuisance or disturbance on NHS premises could result in prosecution. (NHS 2009, 9)

The responsibility for patients and prospective patients of the NHS then is to manage oneself and one's susceptibility to disease, to manage one's compliance in relation to advice and one's comportment on NHS premises.

The coalition government formed after the UK election on 6 May 2010 wasted little time in underscoring responsibility as a key theme in its policymaking. In the first key policy document 'Freedom, Fairness and Responsibility' (Cabinet Office 2010, 8), David Cameron and Nick Clegg outlined an ambition to 'build the free, fair and responsible society we want to see'.

Moreover, in doing so they sought to create 'a stronger society, a smaller state, and power and responsibility in the hands of every citizen' (Cabinet Office 2010, 8).

From the outset, it was clear that a key part of this process of foregrounding responsibility involved devolving it to individuals. David Cameron's aims were to redistribute responsibility from 'the elite in Whitehall to the man and woman in the street' (McVeigh 2010, 33). As the new leaders said later in 'Freedom, Fairness and Responsibility': 'We need an ambitious strategy to prevent ill-health which harnesses innovative techniques to help people take responsibility for their own health' (Cabinet Office 2010, 28).

Shortly thereafter, the new secretary of state for health, Andrew Lansley, unveiled a new white paper that described the ambitions of the new administration as

> to enable people to have greater control over their care and support so they can enjoy maximum independence and responsibility for their own lives. (Department of Health 2010, 10)

And:

> In return for greater choice and control, patients should accept responsibility for the choices they make, concordance with treatment programmes and the implications for their lifestyle. (Department of Health 2010, 16)

This was put more bluntly by health minister Anne Milton, as reported in the *Daily Telegraph* (29 July 2010) by Andrew Bloxham:

> Doctors should call people 'fat' rather than 'obese' to make it clear that they needed to lose weight, a health minister said yesterday. Anne Milton, a Conservative, said the term 'obese' distanced people from the problem and that calling them fat would encourage 'personal responsibility'. She said many NHS professionals were worried that if they called people 'fat' they might cause offence but she insisted that anyone with such a weight problem needed to know. 'If I look in the mirror and think I am obese I think I am less worried than if I think I am fat,' said Mrs Milton after the publication of the Coalition's public health plans. 'You cannot do it for them. People have to have the information.' (Bloxham 2010, 10)

In this view, the nomenclature deployed can force responsibility upon people. The responsible citizen will adjust their body mass index as a result of the expert advice. Whether people are called obese or fat, what is clear on both sides of the debate is that the question of how much one weighs is a matter for the government. To say this might appear banal yet it is this aspect that seems to us most extraordinary. How did this private matter become a topic for government intervention at all? So great is the adherence of the coalition government to this kind of interventionist approach that it has appointed Kris Murrin, presenter of a series of television programmes called *Honey, We're Killing The Kids*, as an adviser and head of David Cameron's 'implementation unit'.

As the reader might suspect by now, the scientific case for government sponsored interventions to control weight is somewhat ambiguous. The customary advice is to maintain a body mass index (weight in kilogrammes divided by height in metres squared) of between 18 and 25. Yet a good deal of evidence suggests that people who are 'overweight' with body mass indices between 25 and 30 enjoy better health than those who are within the recommended range. Health risks increase noticeably for those with body mass indices over 30 and especially over 35, but up to that point the health value of lowering one's weight is debatable (Flegal and Graubard 2009; Flegal, Graubard et al. 2005; Gronniger 2005). Our point here is not to suggest that the work of Flegal et al. should be epistemologically privileged over and above popular health advice in any simple sense. As will become apparent later in this book, we are often critical of supposedly scientific knowledge and the means by which it is generated and promulgated. What we are doing is pointing out the disconnections that exist between the advice and the science which purportedly underlies it.

The interesting question is what the popular advice and government intervention is for and what purpose it serves. One answer drawn from our discussion of neoliberalism above is that the relationship between people and themselves, their bodies and their dietary habits has become a matter for mediation by the state and by public health communication experts. The earlier forms of experience of appetite and exercise, whereby one might eat if one was hungry or if one's companions were eating, or whether one might be physically active for pleasure or because of one's employment, have been superseded by a process of governance. The individual is responsibilized, certainly – food intake, salt intake and the like are matters which we are enjoined to self-regulate in the interests of taking responsibility for our health – yet at the same time we are acclimatized to a high degree of governmental intervention in the relationship with ourselves and those around us.

This is the key dilemma or contradiction with which we shall be concerned in this volume. On the one hand virtues of independence, responsibility, resourcefulness and self-investment are celebrated, yet at the same time we are enjoined to live our lives through a matrix of advice and governmentality in which we are continually urged to mistrust our own judgement and our involvement in organic and spontaneous social relationships, and we are admonished that our conduct should be guided by governmentally sanctioned expertise.

Conclusion

In this chapter we have sketched out how some of the key concepts which were once conceptualized in terms of rights are increasingly seen as involving responsibilities too, especially since, as many commentators have noted, the state is seeking to restrict its formal responsibility for citizens' welfare in a number of spheres. Whilst once neoliberalism might have been about economics, and premised on an ethos of 'small government' and liberalized opportunities for entrepreneurs and investors, it has more recently come to embrace desired modes of conduct in enterprising, self-responsible citizens. This, if anything, has been enhanced by the difficulties faced in the business environment since 2008 and the fact that many states have increased, rather than decreased, their involvement in their economies in efforts to stabilize the crises. The sphere of personal conduct is managed increasingly via the maxims of individualism, minimal state involvement and the valorization of supposedly self-reliant entrepreneurial dispositions on the part of individuals.

The process of responsibilization involves a reformulation of governance, away from what was once called the 'legislative conceit', whereby attempts were made to govern through legislation which prohibited or mandated particular courses of action. Instead, responsibilization involves establishing and consolidating desirable courses of action through manifestations of knowledge or expertise. Once informed, so the logic goes, the citizen should be rendered trustworthy and predictable, and their capacity for self-management as prudent and rational citizens will be increased. The current generation of policymakers have sought to place responsibility centre stage in their discussions of society and social reform. Indeed, this has been styled by Baroness Sayeeda Warsi as a 'responsibility revolution' (Cabinet Office 2011).

As we shall see in subsequent chapters, however, the situation is more complex and more pervasive. The assemblage of mechanisms to encourage and enforce responsibility is not solely concerned with abandoning citizens. It is, as we shall see, also concerned with advising them, shaping them and applying a variety of civil and penal sanctions through an increasingly dense framework of legislation to enforce responsibility in situations where individuals persist in flouting the advice and guidance given. One of the areas in which this framework of responsibilization is most obvious is that of health and it is to this that we will turn in the next chapter.

Chapter Three

INDIVIDUALISM IN HEALTHCARE

Introduction: The Language of Biopower

In this chapter, we will explore some aspects of debates on health and health policy where they pertain to the notion of responsibility. Our discussion of the discourses of individualism and responsibility in healthcare will pay particular attention to language. The importance of this hinges on the notion that there is a dialectical relationship between society and discourse such that society (and culture) are both shaped by and simultaneously constitute discourse (Titscher, Meyer et al. 2000; Thapar-Bjorket and Morgan 2010). The centrality of language is underscored by Peters (2001, 59) when he observes:

> The state has only been able to begin the process of writing itself out of its traditional responsibilities concerning the welfare state through twin strategies of a greater individualisation of society and the responsibilisation of individuals and families.

The role of language and means of communicating on policy and the broader impress of power has been particularly well explored in work on 'biopower'. This phrase was originally used by Foucault to describe the 'explosion of numerous and diverse techniques for achieving the subjugations of bodies and the control of populations' (Foucault 1978, 140).
Biopower serves to

> bring into view a field comprised of more or less rationalized attempts to intervene upon the vital characteristics of human existence. The vital characteristics of human beings, as living creatures who are born, mature, inhabit a body that can be trained and augmented, and then sicken and die. And the vital characteristics of collectivities or populations composed of such living beings. (Rabinow and Rose 2006, 196–7)

As seen by Foucault, Rabinow and Rose, biopower does not predominantly operate through coercion – although we may see coercive elements in it – but through the normalization and medicalization of conduct. Illness comes to be seen as an outward sign of neglect of one's corporeal self – a condition considered as shameful, dirty or irresponsible. As this becomes sedimented into common sense among policymakers and the population as a whole, 'historically entrenched institutionalized forms of social control discipline bodies' through 'laws, medical interventions, social institutions, ideologies and even structures of feeling' (Bourgois 2000, 167). Authors who have focused on biopower have identified shifts in the way in which health and social care services are framed and delivered, as well as changes in the mission of institutions, ideas and practices of 'advanced' or *neo*liberalism.

Welfarism and the Growth of Governmentality

In the period after the Second World War, policymakers in developed nations typically espoused a 'welfarist' political rationality which emphasized state, institutional and collective responsibility for the care of individual citizens. Under conditions of neoliberalism, a political rationality has surfaced in which rational, independent and entrepreneurial citizens are increasingly responsible for the 'care of the self' (Petersen 1997). In connection with this, there have been movements toward non-collective, low cost solutions to the 'problem' of growing welfare budgets, a deinstitutionalization of healthcare, privatization of services, adoption of user pays models and promotion of more active forms of citizenship (Moore 2009; Nettleton and Bunton 1995). In terms of the public services, the implications of this have been characterized by Kemshall (2002, 132):

> In advanced liberal societies governmentality is displaced to the microdomain of individual and locale, with the residual role of welfare agencies constituted as facilitating prudential choices through the provision of expert knowledge and in the provision of 'rational choices' for the individual.

Hence, the exhortations for the citizen to manage their own conduct in relation to health have both a fiscal and a moral quality. Individuals are exhorted to become virtuous biocitizens through strategies for managing risk at a population level and through an 'individualizing focus' (Bunton 1997, 229). This has also involved the creation of what Bernstein (2001) terms a 'pedagogized society'. In Bernstein's view, a good deal of the social and economic business of contemporary societies involves a kind of pedagogy such that a process of learning takes place through the home, the mass media, the workplace and increasingly through electronic media. In this way, the population is taught about health and its associated risks through instructional and regulatory pedagogies (Evans, Davies et al. 2004). Thus, expertise is brought to bear on the individuals' conduct often in the guise of support aimed at minimizing the risks of contemporary living. The healthy citizen is thus part of a project to imbue themselves with responsibility to

> ceaselessly maintain and improve her or his own health by using a whole range of measures. To do this she or he is increasingly expected to take note of and act upon the recommendations of a whole range of 'experts' and 'advisors' located in a range of diffuse institutional and cultural sites. (Bunton and Burrows 1995, 208)

In the case of weight control and the avoidance of obesity, Halse (2007) suggests that 'personal responsibility for one's weight is constituted as care for oneself and for others and therefore as a moral and ethical duty to wider society'. Whilst, in most circumstances, there is a degree of voluntarism where compliance with advice is concerned, there may also be more materially obtrusive elements. For example, Kmietowicz (2011) reports that referrals for elective surgery in Hertfordshire have dropped 'dramatically' as a result of general practitioners referring patients who smoke or whose body mass index is over 30 to smoking cessation or weight loss interventions, rather than surgery itself. This illustrates the slippage between choice, responsibility and compulsion noted by Petersen, Davies et al. (2010).

The slippage between prudent, voluntary control of one's bodily deportment and more coercive measures can be illustrated also by recent legal cases reported in the news media. For example, regarding sexual health, in February 2010 German popular singer Nadja Benassia was charged with causing bodily harm because she had unprotected sex with four men between 2000 and 2004, allegedly without telling them that she was HIV positive (BBC 2010a). When arrested in April 2009, it was reported that the authorities judged that the 'risk of repetition' was such that she was held in custody. However after ten days she was released and faced trial in August 2010, charged with grievous bodily harm on the ex-partner who subsequently became HIV positive and attempted aggravated assault on two other partners (Yeoman 2009). On 26 August 2010, Benassia was found guilty on one count of causing grievous bodily harm and two counts of attempted bodily harm and was given a two year suspended sentence (BBC 2010b).

Although high profile, this is not an isolated case. Estimates suggest that 600 people across 40 countries have been convicted of offences in relation to HIV, even though such cases rarely involve deliberate transmission (J. Smith 2010). What is important from our point of view is that such charges can be brought at all, that one can be legally held responsible or accountable for the actions not only of oneself but for the notional activities of the microbial life to which one plays host. Whilst provisions have existed under English law to hold someone legally responsible for passing on sexually transmitted infections since 1861, high profile cases have become a much more conspicuous feature of the legal landscape more recently. What is interesting is why this process of responsibilization is happening now rather than, for example, at times when the prevalence of transmissible diseases – especially sexually transmitted infections – was much higher. In late modernity we are uniquely responsible for managing the risks that our bodies may present to others. Allied to this, as Squire (2010) notes, there has been a redefinition of HIV as a long-term chronic condition, which, like diabetes, heart disease and certain cancers, confers particular lifestyle obligations on its sufferers to live self-regulating, healthy lives. In tandem with this, there are a variety of legislative sanctions for those left behind in the new climate of responsible HIV citizenship.

A similar process can be seen at work in discussions of passive smoking where this might affect children. Chair of the UK Royal College of General Practitioners, Professor Steve Field, wrote an article in the *Observer* in the summer of 2010, claiming that:

> I believe that parents who smoke in cars carrying small children are committing a form of child abuse; I suppose the same people also smoke at home in front of their children. Evidence from the US indicates that more young children are killed by parental smoking than by all unintentional injuries combined. (Field 2010, 25)

We shall consider Field's comments in relation to the responsibilization process in a moment. For the moment, let us note that the benefits of reducing passive smoking are not entirely clear-cut or decisive. Expert evidence collected by the House of Lords Economic Affairs Committee (House of Lords 2006) for its 2006 report tended to the view that the risks from passive smoking are 'uncertain, and unlikely to be large'. Some large scale studies have reported only limited and non-significant effects associated with passive smoking on heart disease and lung cancer, the effects of which may be 'considerably weaker than generally believed' (Enstrom and Kabat 2003). The point is not to make definitive pronouncements on the risk of passive smoking but rather to highlight the purchase which representations of such hazards readily gain and their implications for individual conduct. Once the deleterious effects of passive smoking are assimilated into the regime of truth they 'cannot be intelligibly questioned' (Ungar and Bray 2005, 5). Representations of risk take on a life of their own far in excess of their purported scientific basis (Kabat 2008).

Our concern with passive smoking has to do with the process of responsibilization because, like the HIV in the example earlier, it makes the individual accountable for the consequences of their actions for others. Rather than one's microbes, one is responsible in this case for one's second or even third hand smoke particles. It is the purported effect on others that provides the rationale for the legislation facilitating the blurring of the distinction between public and private. Irrespective of the strength of the effect of passive smoking on health, any proposed legislation and the debate surrounding it relies on the image of the smoker themselves as a particularly culpable source of environmental contamination.

The focus in this chapter, and in this book more generally, will be on issues where links between the management of conduct in practical contexts – health, housing, justice, therapy and so on – and the notions of governmentality and responsibilization are clearly visible. We will be focusing on areas where there is, in the scientific literature, more room for debate and scepticism, for it is here that the processes of governmentality and the regulation of conduct may be more clearly seen as relatively autonomous processes. There are a variety of examples where the actuarial risks are far more clear-cut and a utilitarian, social contract rationale for legislation might be elaborated more persuasively. These might include the risks from first hand smoke from one's own smoking, legislation concerned to regulate drink driving, the possession and use of firearms, the mandatory provision of fire exits in public buildings and the like. Whilst processes of legislation, persuasion and regulation are apparent in these cases, our interest is in instances where the question of scientifically estimated risk or the apportionment of culpability is more ambiguous or debatable; where public health initiatives, for example, have a more tenuous link with evidence or where there is at least room for informed scepticism. It is in these cases that governmentality and the allied processes of individualization and responsibilization have been let off the leash. It is where they have developed a measure of autonomy from the evidence base taken as a whole that they are at their most conspicuous and, from our point of view, most interesting.

Ideas, practices and forms of self-management derive, in part, from discourses of evidence, but examples where the evidence base is more debatable highlight the importance of examining the origins and the deployment of present day discourses of responsibility where health is concerned. In doing this, following Maynard (1988, 318) it may be possible to understand how professionals, policymakers and legislators 'procedurally produce and experience forms of "trouble" that may emerge as problems and deviance' on the part of the citizenry. In addition to changes being brought about through the legislature and policy documents, Buttny (2004, 2) alerts us, via the pronouncements of the great and good in the popular media, to the way that in all these sources 'problems can be told through various actions such as narratives, claims, descriptions, accusations, complaints and the like'. Problems can be accounted for through telling stories which exemplify individual citizens' doings and non-doings (Hall 1997).

The presently ascendant neoliberal political stances help to foreground the citizen's personal responsibility. The responsibility in question is demanded especially of those who are marginalized or, in contemporary parlance, 'socially excluded' (Jordan and Jordan 2000; Rose 2002). In health, as in other spheres of social life, as Webb (2006, 65) notes '…the socially excluded are offered choice and self-determination, whilst their conduct and patterns of life are simultaneously regulated and normalized'. Moore (2009) describes in his study of injecting drug users in an Australian city, how clients are expected to take responsibility to plan their affairs. In some cases, the clients adopted the language of service provision themselves, talking of their 'risk taking' behaviour or their failure to control their 'impulses'. In less abject cases it remains the individual who is enjoined to modify their errant conduct – smokers, those deemed overweight or people who are alleged to take insufficient exercise, for example.

Self-Imposed and Self-Managed Risks: Triumph of the Will

A corollary of this emphasis on conduct is the emphasis on the interior space of the self as a key arena for change. Attitudes, values, decision making and choice are formulated as the underlying machinery behind conduct and it is to these variables that a good deal of the discourse of health is directed.

Historians of public health often point to the so-called 'Lalonde Report' named after the then minister of national health and welfare in Canada, Marc Lalonde (Lalonde 1974; Berridge 2009). This is often cited as one of the first government documents in the contemporary era to make extensive reference to the importance of self-imposed risks in the management of public health. It made explicit reference to the importance of 'lifestyle hazards which contribute heavily to the frequency of sickness and death' (Lalonde 1974, 8). Lifestyle, Lalonde said, 'consists of the aggregation of decisions by individuals which affect their health and over which they more or less have control… Personal decisions and habits that are bad, from a health point of view, create self-imposed risks' (Lalonde 1974, 32). He pointed to the 'grisly litany of the more destructive lifestyle habits and their consequences' (1974, 16). Whilst lifestyle was only one of the foci of this report, it signalled an important opening up of focus in which the individual and his or her decisions were concerned, and this helped to consolidate the process of responsibilization for one's own health.

In the UK, this agenda was underlined by the government publication of 'Prevention and Health: Everybody's Business (Department of Health and Social Security 1976). The phrase 'everybody's business' implied individual and communal responsibility rather than the previous emphasis on collective, state mandated solutions or clinical facilities and services.

'Choosing Health' (Department of Health 2004, 3) was explicitly premised on the notion that to understand health one needed to understand the choices people made: 'Health is inextricably linked to the way people live their lives and the opportunities available to choose health in the communities where they live'. Whilst there is a focus on geographic and socioeconomic differences in health, this is seen as being because people in straitened economic circumstances

> are often less likely to think about the consequences of everyday choices about diet, exercise, smoking and sexual behaviour on their long-term health, or to take up the childhood immunisation and health screening programmes that provide protection against diseases that can kill or cause serious long-term ill-health. (Department of Health 2004, 8)

Therefore, it is through the medium of choices and people's inability to exercise healthy choices that dire socioeconomic conditions are seen to have an effect on health. Rather than poverty harming us directly, it is through our own failure to choose to take steps to maintain a healthy lifestyle that its invidious effects are accomplished. Choice is central to a good deal of policy discourse at a national level in the UK, functioning as an image that structures governmental orientations to policy (Clarke, Newman et al. 2007). It has often been contrasted with the so-called 'old' model of public services based on the 'one size fits all' principle (Office of Public Service Reform 2002, 13). Building on discourses of choice that were a legacy from the previous Conservative administration that had championed campaigns such as the 'right to buy' council housing and parental 'choice' in education, New Labour presented its reforms of public services by promulgating a consumerist or marketized conception of choice as an organizing principle (Clarke, Newman et al. 2007).

The present day idea of the self as a means of mediating the relationship between health and illness and the mind and the body can be traced to some of the significant currents of thought in the nineteenth century. To a number of Victorian medical thinkers, for example J. C. Prichard and John Haslam, the person's 'will' served to mediate between the mind and the body. If the will were to degenerate this would inevitably lead to insanity and moral decay. In this view, the will served as a bulwark against the bodily passions and served to protect the mind's rationality. Prichard describes the symptoms of insanity in which the 'disordered condition of the mind displays itself in a want of self-government, in continual excitement, and unusual expression of strong feelings' (Prichard 1837, 25). These problems were taken to represent the failure of the will to control the body and its impulses. Implicit in this perspective is the idea that passions and intense emotions are linked to insanity, especially if they escape the governance of the will. These physical passions which were often seen as somehow bestial and sexual were able to gain control over the disordered mind. In this Victorian conception both madness and a disposition to satisfy one's 'impulses' were linked to physical and moral lapse.

The role of the will becomes even more significant once its connection to the political mindset of the era is explored. Writing in 1884, Maudsley asserts that 'a loss of power over the thoughts, feelings, and acts is an essential fact of anarchy' (Maudsley 1884, 284–5). In this way it was established that the will served a key role in regulating an individual but also in governing society itself. A lapse of the will causes disorder and the 'loss of power' that comes with individual madness or moral degeneration and with it the undermining of fundamental social notions of disciplined and restrained conduct.

This kind of emphasis on the will and the power of thought, especially positive thinking and personal power, were popularized through the works of a number of writers affiliated with what was called the New Thought movement in the US. One of its well known proponents, Phineas Parkhurst Quimby (1802–1866), proposed that illness originates in the mind as a result of erroneous beliefs and that healing involved opening one's mind to God's wisdom. Another member of the New Thought movement was William Walker Atkinson (1862–1932), who emphasized the power of the will to control thoughts in his book *Thought Vibration* (1906). Once this necessity has been mastered and we are able to declaim that we are full of courage and that we desire things calmly and confidently then, via the so-called law of attraction, the things that we desire such as health, wealth and love, will come to us through the power of thought alone. The discourse of self-help is, as Illouz (2008) stated, a 'political technology of the self'. Self-help, from the nineteenth century to the present day, is more than just a hermeneutic device that assists individuals in making sense of their condition. It also is a cultural device by means of which we can tap into and channel complex cultural and affective apparatuses. These can make intelligible and desirable particular patterns of thought and forms of conduct, and afford new kinds of individual and collective action on the self and on communities.

Throughout the twentieth century this form of self-help thinking – that success originates in the mindset rather than in material opportunities – was elaborated further by a variety of popular writers. Among them was Napoleon

Hill (1883–1970), author of a variety of self-help books, notably *Think And Grow Rich* (1937). Dale Carnegie, (1888–1955) author of *How To Win Friends And Influence People* (1936), emphasized self-confidence and a constructive attitude. The focus of much of this work was to carve out an interior space that the individual could usefully work upon to achieve wealth, personal fulfilment and health. The furniture, as it were, in this space differed little between the different proponents of New Thought or self-help, and similar themes can be seen in many contemporary self-help books.

To take just one example, the popular volume *The Secret* by Rhonda Byrne (2006), suggests that by visualizing wealth, abundance and health these will be attracted to the reader by means of the 'law of attraction'. For example, if one wishes to lose weight one needs to avoid the company of overweight people and instead switch one's mind to one's own perfect body. Ehrenreich (2009) notes that this kind of approach gives credence to a whole range of superstitions and prejudicial thinking that was challenged by the Enlightenment. Victim blaming, believing that failure is the result of not trying hard enough or not visualizing success with sufficient confidence, is substituted for a more thoroughgoing engagement with the problems that result in poverty and ill health.

Byrne's *The Secret* reprises the popular advice of Wallace D. Wattles (1860–1911), who, in a book entitled *The Science of Getting Rich* (1910), proposed a similar system to attract abundance by means of will power and mastery over the self. The notion of abundance plays a key role in Covey's *The Seven Habits of Highly Effective People* (1989) in which an 'abundance mentality' is associated with high self-worth and security. Yet at the same time, responsibility and self-help has been urged most strongly on the very poorest in developed nations (Schmidtz and Goodin 1998), where the likelihood of attracting abundance by means of thought alone is least likely. What is interesting from our point of view is not the way that these apparently superstitious ways of thinking about the self in the world are at odds with more sober assessments of one's chances, or the way in which they contradict a good deal of Enlightenment rationality. Our interest is to do with how these instruments of culture help to transform and give shape and form to personal and social experience. Rather than propose a 'better' way of managing health or organizing society, our interest is in thinking through how the culture of responsibility works, how it has been sedimented into common sense and how it reproduces itself successfully. From writing and publishing, gathering together to support one another and share ideas and by providing a common language of self-understanding, self-help has for a century and a half provided ways of sharing and collectivizing experiences, communicating them with others and organizing shared activity in significant domains of human experience.

For example, as McGrath, Jordens et al. (2006) argue, the notion of thinking positively in the face of illness is particularly widely and uncritically accepted. This may, they say, reflect popular beliefs about the relationship between mind and body, the nature of health and disease and the obligation that sick people have to help themselves and discover positive experiences in illness (Schroevers, Kraaij et al. 2010). As we have mentioned, a further source of this notion has been the influence of popular psychology self-help literature. Added to this, we can trace the popular perceptions of complementary and alternative medicine. This has informed public perceptions of the mechanisms of disease such that the attitude of the suffering individual is seen as being particularly culpable.

Responsibility, Policy and Employability

The discourses of policymakers and prominent intellectuals do not all urge responsibility in the same way or to the same effect. The calls present in politicians' speeches reported in the popular press for a 'responsibility revolution' differ from the more measured tones of policy documents, and think tank discourse is often different again. The subtlety of this mélange of voices is illustrated when we examine how clients of public services are conceptualized across this range of sources.

The *Marmot Review* (Marmot 2010) was published as a result of a two year investigation by Michael Marmot and colleagues into health inequalities, discussing also policy implications and issues which will come to the fore in the future. This is clearly a different document from many others in the policy field where responsibility is concerned. It commences with a stirring quote from poet Pablo Neruda – 'Rise up with me against the organization of misery'. Examining the text for mentions of responsibility discloses that the term overwhelmingly occurs in relation to collective entities – the government or government departments, civic institutions, employers and the like. The report argues that individual empowerment requires social action (Marmot 2010, 34). There are, however, some areas where notions of responsibility pertaining to the individual were underscored. The promotion of 'active engagement on the part of clients of public services' was key to providing a

> springboard for enhancing the lives of users who might be marginalised or stigmatised, enabling them to exercise greater degrees of control and responsibility. (Marmot 2010, 159)

On the other hand, the Department for Work and Pensions (2008) green paper 'No One Written Off' is subtitled 'Reforming Welfare to Reward

Responsibility' and is explicitly concerned with promoting and sustaining the ideals of neoliberal citizenship discussed earlier:

> Research has shown that being in work generally improves people's health. Increasingly, doctors agree that remaining in work is often in their patients' best interests and should be seen as an indicator of a successful clinical outcome. (Department for Work and Pensions 2008, 31)

The idea of being 'fit for work' and the notion of health assessments focusing on ability rather than impairments – so-called 'fit notes' – originally proposed by Dame Carol Black, was endorsed. 'Paid work is the route to independence, health and well-being for most people' (Department for Work and Pensions 2008, 25).

Health is itself a metaphor for a broader selection of traits that concern one's effectiveness as a job seeker. In 'No One Written Off', a frequent 'skills health check' is recommended – often under powers of compulsion – to ensure that the project of the self as an employable entity is proceeding apace. This process looks set to continue under the coalition government elected in the UK in May 2010 as plans are formulated to reduce the purported burden on the public purse. This stance is being further consolidated by some leading members of the medical profession itself. Professor Steve Field, in his role as chair of the Royal College of General Practitioners, described how he had detected with the 2010 change of government an even greater emphasis 'for individuals to take more personal responsibility for their health and the health of their children'. Moreover:

> Parents really do need to take more responsibility...this should start even before conception... Women who want to conceive, or are newly pregnant, need to take more responsibility as part of their commitment to the child they hope to carry. (Field 2010, 25)

This transformation in liberal social governance in which individuals are implicated in their roles as citizens and family members represents a shift of emphasis from social responsibilities toward individualized, private responsibilities (Petersen, Davies et al. 2010). Whilst this shift focuses upon how the individual should conduct themselves, it also reflects the supervention of a broader neoliberal governmental style of thinking about and acting upon problems, that Ilcan (2009) calls 'privatizing responsibility'. At a time of growing financial austerity in public services in many nations, this privatization of responsibility has involved a move away from a view of citizenship based upon collectively respected social rights (Molz 2005).

This has undermined an earlier welfarist position in which the systemically disadvantaged and their advocates could argue for the state to regulate and avert the structural undermining of individual and collective wellbeing (Brodie 2007).

Instead, the focus now is not so much on investment in capital projects to alleviate deprivation, but rather on legislation aimed at the regulation of conduct. The pricing of alcoholic drinks and tobacco products, the regulation of advertising, the development of campaigns to modify eating habits and the like are at the very heart of austerity policy discourse. This accelerates and augments the trend towards redefining citizenship in terms of entrepreneurial responsibilities on the part of individuals themselves in terms of how they respond to the governance, legislative shifts and expert mediated advice. The responsible citizen, of course, is the one who addresses his or her errant conduct and reshapes themselves in terms of the current expertise.

This advice and expertise concerning the ideals of healthful conduct towards which the individual should aspire does not come from a single source. The tasks of governance have been devolved towards a variety of non-government agencies, autonomous bodies and, as suggested by the example of Steve Field, to professional organizations. Where policy or legislation is enacted by governments it is backed by 'expertise' granting it a degree of moral or electoral authority. Therefore as Ilcan (2009, 208) says:

> Privatizing responsibility is neither a homogeneous or tightly knit structure or arrangement nor a model of cause and effect. Instead, it comprises diverse elements, shapes forms of conduct, and takes part in various forms of governing.

Yet there are a number of overarching pervasive effects of this kind of policy. The rationality of the responsible citizen themselves is supplanted by the pre-digested advice and expertise which accompanies policy. In this kind of regime it is not up to the citizen to seek out evidence and evaluate the merits of different courses of action or to make moral choices in terms of how she or he seeks to live their lives, but rather to 'choose' on the basis of the advice they are given. This obviates debate, bypasses exploration of possibly conflicting strands of evidence and avoids the potentially problematic and challenging situation that might ensue if sceptical scientific literacy were more democratically distributed. Instead active, responsible individuals are enjoined to make choices, pursue preferences and seek to maximize the quality of their lives inasmuch as they correspond with the advice that they are given.

Interiorizing Health

Ensuring compliance with health education and advice has helped to consolidate new spheres of expertise, research and practice. The proliferation of focus on the individual as an actor in the rituals of health and a guardian of his or her own destiny in the health sphere has occurred in tandem with a research and policy focus on such matters as health behaviour, health beliefs and a wealth of features of the interior landscape such as self-esteem, self-efficacy as well as an array of cognitive and attitudinal factors. This is accompanied by assertions from the shield bearers of health psychology that health behaviours are currently estimated to account for about 40 per cent of premature mortality (McGinnis, Williams-Russo et al. 2002). By 2010, the UK's Cabinet Office Behavioural Insight Team felt able to assert that 'behavioural and lifestyle factors are thought to be major contributors in half of all deaths' (Cabinet Office 2010, 6).

In tandem with this, epidemiology has focused on individual 'lifestyle' factors such as smoking status, weight and diet, to subvert earlier conceptions of inequality based on socioeconomic status and differences originating in wealth and resources. Lifestyle itself is a health commodity, and degree courses are taught in how it might be cultivated and managed. In illness the patient is exhorted to remain 'positive' in the face of assaults from disease and iatrogenic problems arising from medical practice itself. Health psychology has made extensive use of notions which stress the potential of the individual to control their state of wellness with concepts of self-efficacy, locus of control and self-esteem being assiduously measured in relation to health education and healthcare initiatives. These measures of a person's sense of control over their health are addressed in the hope of detecting factors which may enhance or lower compliance with treatment regimes or expert advice. Early work suggested that an internal locus of control – a sense that events in one's life are under one's own control – was associated with greater compliance with advice and treatment recommendations (Wallston and Wallston 1978). More recently the picture is a little more complicated, but those who believe that health is largely a matter of chance rather than something that can be vouchsafed by their own exertions engage in rather less desirable health behaviour (Grotz, Hapk et al. 2011). The more we have a sense that health is under our control, the more likely we are to do what we are told.

The work of health promoters, lifestyle experts and health educators has opened up a particular kind of space in the minds of the public for investigation and scrutiny. It is as if health were a consequence of particular kinds of attitudinal and cognitive factors. To give a flavour of this kind of thinking, let us consider the Transtheoretical Model of Change, a model that has gained a great deal of purchase on the discipline of health psychology and is claimed to inform a good many interventions to promote health behaviour change. The Transtheoretical Model (Prochaska and DiClemente 1983; Prochaska, DiClemente et al. 1992; Prochaska and Velicer 1997) claims to be an 'integrative model of behaviour change' inasmuch as it was designed by its originators to incorporate as much of the existing literature on changes in health behaviour as possible. The term 'transtheroretical' is itself puzzling as the theoretical reach is narrow, concentrating on a restricted suite of psychosocial, cognitive and attitudinal factors.

There are several variants of the model, but they all involve a sequential series of stages in which the citizen seeking to reform their health behaviour goes through. Let us look at a fairly typical account from Rakowski, Fulton et al. (1993) in relation to breast cancer screening via mammography:

1. Pre-contemplation. In this stage the person has no prior record of performing the desired behaviour and no intention of doing so in the foreseeable future.
2. Contemplation. In this stage, the individual is planning to make the desired change soon. They may be aware of the purported advantages but are also aware of the drawbacks.
3. Preparation. Refers to the stage when people are about to take action in the immediate future. These individuals are conjectured to have a plan of action such as joining a health education class, consulting a counsellor, talking to their physician, buying a self-help book or relying on a self-change approach.
4. Action. Refers to the stage where the person has commenced the actions in question and is intending to maintain this course of action in the future. This might include, for example, attending a smoking cessation course, commencing exercise or having had a prior mammogram and planning to have another one in the coming year.
5. Maintenance. Refers to a later stage in the process, where the desired change in conduct is further established and the intention to continue is sustained.
6. Relapse. This item relates to those who have undertaken the desired behaviour in the past but are not presently doing so or are not intending to. This might include women who have had mammograms in the past but are not planning to have one in the coming year, people who have abandoned exercise programmes or have resumed smoking.

The model supposes that there is a logic, order and sequentialization present in the individual's progress through decision and action. In addition, it can readily be seen from this account of the sequence that there are particular tasks for the health professional or educator to perform at each stage in the process to initiate decision making and sustain the desired conduct. Notably absent are any indications that the evidence about the effectiveness or appropriateness of the supposedly desirable course of action may be ambiguous or equivocal or that there may be differing ways of achieving the desired outcome. Absent too is any accounting for socioeconomic or power differences and their impact on health and wealth or their impact on the opportunity to perform the desired behaviour, or the possibility that the desired change in behavior is at odds with the richly contextualized social lives led by the target population (Lindsay 2010). It is perhaps a tribute to the suppleness of the transtheoretical model that even when it appears not to describe or predict change, it may still prevail as an explanation because the participants must have not been at the correct stage in the process of change for the intervention in question (Norcross, Krebs et al. 2011).

The particular interest from our point of view is the kind of assumptions made about language, thought and behaviour. It is assumed that these are relatively orderly – or at least they are if health educators have done their jobs appropriately – and that thinking and decision making are logically prior to conduct. This is not the only or even the majority view of how such a process might work. In many practical contexts language and action have a logic and orderliness that is not readily reducible to cognitive and attitudinal measurement (Potter 2000). Sociological critiques have asserted that the concepts deployed in these kinds of models and accounts of individuals' compliance with advice do not do justice to the complexity and sophistication of lay theorizing about illness (Blaxter 1983; Calnan 1987; Blaxter and Britten 1996; Lindsay 2010; Williams and Calnan 1996). Even within the psychological spaces with which the model is concerned, the scope of health psychological frameworks such as the transtheoretical model are remarkable as much for what they leave out as for what they put in. Ubel and Loewenstein (1997) observe that the psychological feelings associated with medical decision making such as hope, fear and dread are not accounted for.

A number of authors including Radley (1994) and Stainton Rogers (1991) would argue that the way of conceptualizing health found in these kinds of models of health behaviour overemphasizes the role of cognition and underemphasizes the social context within which health related conduct takes place. Indeed 'health' and 'illness' may not be 'fixed entities in the minds of the people concerned' (Radley 1994, 55) and health related cognition is likely not to be consistent, stable and predictive of behaviour in any simple sense.

The question then remains of what these highly selective and specific models of healthcare decision making and behavioural change are serving to do.

According to Trostle (1988) and Britten (2001) the main function is ideological: to provide a framework for doctors to express their ideas about how patients *ought* to behave. Models such as this offer clear justification for attributing blame when patients' actions do not match the expectations placed on them by health professionals (Donovan and Blake 1992; Britten 2001).

The effect of these kinds of frameworks to open up to scrutiny and rearrangement the space inside the citizens' head is aligned with what Anthony Giddens had to say two decades ago about reflexivity:

> The reflexivity of modern social life consists in the fact that social practices are constantly examined and reformed in the light of incoming information about those very practices, thus constitutively altering their character...only in the era of modernity is the revision of convention radicalised to apply (in principle) to all aspects of human life... (Giddens 1990, 38–9)

There are two related aspects to the phenomenon that we are talking about. One is for educators, health promoters and policymakers to see the citizen in terms of interior, cognitive and attitudinal variables which can be adjusted. The second is for people to see themselves as if they were projects upon which they can work via resolutions to reduce drinking, give up smoking, join gyms and health clubs and so on. The tendency to see health in terms of arrangements of the mental architecture encourages a degree of self-scrutiny where health practices and beliefs are concerned and an implication that the responsible citizen will constantly adjust themselves in the light of new information as it is available. The function of these approaches is to encourage and enhance a particular way of thinking about the self. It is a means of making sense of oneself and other citizens under advanced liberalism that foregrounds the role of mental machinery in the processes of health, rather than for example broader social or ideological structures and processes or the practice of politics itself.

In addition to the way in which citizens are hailed by a variety of exhortations to modify their thinking and behaviour in the interests of achieving better health, there are other technologies of the self at work. To return to the themes of the New Thought movement that we described briefly earlier, it is apposite to examine how in the present day we are exhorted to 'think positively'. This is pervasively encouraged, especially in healthcare settings where patients are faced with chronic or life-threatening conditions.

As McGrath, Jordens et al. (2006) note, this may take several forms. In their study of positive thinking in the case of cancer sufferers and carers, they note that two major kinds of benefits are claimed for positive thinking. The first is that positive thinking will enable the sufferer to cope better with the illness and the experience of treatment. The second is that positive thinking will itself contribute to a favourable outcome such that the cancer will be cured or the patient will at least benefit from an extended period of remission. The prospect of these benefits may be appealing to patients and carers as well as to healthcare professionals because they offer the hope that patients can exercise a means of helping themselves. As a number of authors including McGrath, Jordens et al. (2006) and Ehrenreich (2009) point out, these presumed benefits are not supported by the published literature seeking to determine whether there is any effect of positive thinking on morbidity or mortality. There is evidence to suggest that cancer sufferers with an 'optimistic outlook' and a 'fighting spirit' have a better quality of life than those who are pessimistic and feel hopeless (Schou, Ekeberg et al. 2005). Yet this is just as likely to be to do with overlap between the self-report questionnaires used to measure these variables, than optimism causing improved quality of life in any simple sense. In addition, some evidence suggests that thinking positively helps to provide a sense of control in uncertain situations and may reduce the likelihood of depression (Taylor 1983; Link, Robbins et al. 2004). Taylor emphasized the value of 'gaining a sense of mastery' over the disease. An important aspect of 'successful adjustment' is believed to be manifested through 'a belief that a positive attitude would keep the cancer from coming back' (Taylor 1983, 1163).

Such was the belief in the value of positive thinking in cancer patients on the part of some clinicians and researchers that, for example, Greer and colleagues (Greer, Moorey et al. 1992, 675) were at pains to identify and combat 'psychological morbidity' in cancer patients who attained low scores on self-reported 'fighting spirit'. Patients lacking fighting spirit in this study were provided with adjuvant psychological therapy based on cognitive behavioural principles to teach them to replace their 'negative automatic thoughts' with 'a constructive and positive approach to coping with cancer' (Moorey and Greer 1989, 78). They included examples of 'positive self-statements' that patients were recommended to use such as: 'I'm going to beat this'; 'I know the chemotherapy is shrinking my lump'; 'This isn't going to ruin my life' and 'I'm going to get well' (Moorey and Greer 1989, 117).

Yet, for all the emphasis on positive thinking and the assumption that this reflects the contents of a putative interior space in the patient's psychology, the situation may not be so straightforward. As Wilkinson and Kitzinger (2000, 797) say,

'thinking positive' functions not as an accurate report of an internal cognitive state, but rather as a conversational idiom, characterised by vagueness and generality, and summarising a socially normative moral requirement.

The emphasis on positive thinking in the face of serious illness represents not a panacea which changes one's actuarial chances of survival, but a means of organizing and disciplining the ill citizen. They are 'technologies imbued with aspirations for the shaping of conduct in the hope of producing certain desired effects and averting certain undesired ones' (Rose 2002, 52). People's statements about health and illness are not an expression of their inner thoughts on the subject, but rather the mobilization of culturally available explanations. The stories that they tell and the explanations that they deploy occur in a context of differentiated powers, such that the authority of some regimes such as medicine, psychology or public health complement the work of the state per se often through the exercise of expertise. This differentiation into a multiplicity of different agencies, addressing different facets of conduct and deploying different measures was anticipated by Hunt and Wickham (1994, 76), when they said that 'governmentality is the dramatic expansion in the scope of government, featuring an increase in the number and size of the governmental calculation mechanisms'.

Emphases on the care of the self, health related thinking, attitudes, conduct and on positive thinking in the face of life-threatening illness represent the implication of a variety of agencies, professional groupings and spheres of human activity in the 'governmental calculation process'. In addition, the relentless interiority of much theory and research in health education and health psychology has facilitated the growth of thinking about how individuals should assemble an account of their intentions, actions and future conduct. This involves citizens becoming increasingly responsibilized by encouraging them to see social risks such as ill health not as the responsibility of the state, but as instead lying in the domain for which the individual is responsible and reconfiguring it as a matter of 'self care' (Lemke 2001, 201). As du Gay (2000, 75) has observed:

> Embedded in these contemporary programmes and strategies for the reformulation of social governance is a particular ethic of personhood – a view of what persons are and what they should be allowed to be.

Conclusion: Interiorized Health and the Apotheosis of Expertise

In this chapter, we have explored how the individual is enjoined to be a healthy, entrepreneurial citizen across a range of sites in policy and therapeutic contexts and how the individual's health is formulated as a matter of self-care. Yet at the heart of this there lies a contradiction. If the healthy, responsible behaviour of the self is based on the advice and technical know-how of experts, this tends to tie the individual into a conception of their tasks as a moral being which effectively deskills and shackles them, while seeming to raise their status to that of autonomous citizens. This is made feasible because the 'public objectives for the good health and good order of the social body' are configured so that they appear to have been brought into alignment 'with the desire of individuals for health and well-being' (Rose 2002, 74). Rather, 'individuals are addressed on the assumption that they want to be healthy and enjoined to freely seek out the ways of living most likely to promote their own health' (Rose 2002, 86–7). Therefore, the promotion of health is a technology of self for 'evaluating and acting upon ourselves so that the police, the guards and the doctors do not have to do so' (Cruikshank 1996, 234). It would be too easy to propose a simple dichotomy, such that there is society, the health establishment or government on one side, and the individual on the other, and society imposes its will upon the individual. It is rather that the predominant ways of talking about individuals, the forms of social organization and discourse help to afford the potential for certain kinds of individual actualization and vice versa.

The kind of liberty that is facilitated and the kinds of freedoms that individuals are encouraged to manifest are closely governed so as to be compatible with the tenets of neoliberalism. If neoliberal government is to achieve its goals, a particular kind of consciousness is demanded of individual citizens such that they come to recognize and act upon themselves as both free and responsible (Rose 2002, 68). Thus, neoliberalism must work to create the social reality that it proposes already exists. The mentality of government 'is not pure, neutral knowledge that simply re-presents the governing reality' (Lemke 2001, 191). Under conditions of neoliberalism there are attempts to combine reductions in state health and welfare provision to the increasing deployment of technologies of the self so that citizens come to have the appearance of free, enterprising, autonomous individuals.

This does not mean that individuals are mere putty in the hands of policymakers, think tank specialists or dominant economic interests. Individuals do not inevitably rise to the challenges to be more responsible or enterprising, as the limited uptake of a great many health and wellbeing initiatives has shown. Indeed, it is precisely because the public is often recalcitrant in the face of these urgings that they are repeated. It is to explore the inner workings of the citizen that the sometimes complex and technical-sounding explorations of the individual's decision making processes are undertaken, perhaps with a sequential, rational choice scheme, such as Prochaska's transtheoretical model, or the kinds of theorizing about half submerged affective and cognitive processes that is favoured by the Cabinet

Office Behavioural Insight Team. This brave new 'orthopaedics of the soul' is occasioned precisely because simply telling people what to do has so far had limited effect. This discourse of the healthy, responsible citizen is significant not because of its minatory power, but because such thinking opens up new ways of theorizing about citizens, talking about them and conjuring new forms of political selfhood into being.

Chapter Four

ENLISTING, MEASURING
AND SHAPING THE INDIVIDUAL IN
HEALTHCARE POLICY AND PRACTICE

Introduction

As we have seen in the previous chapter, notions of individualism apparent in healthcare are increasingly inflected in a way that is consonant with neoliberal politics and the tendencies towards responsibilization as described. The idea of citizens or patients as rational consumers is coming to the fore as they are depicted in the popular media and policy as choosing between treatment options, hospitals and healthcare organizations or even choosing to have operations abroad. An ever greater variety of elective procedures are available to those who can afford them, and the idea of the patient as an entrepreneur, consumer or rational economic agent is driven ever further into service provision across a variety of service areas. In addition, it is increasingly possible to detect consumerist discourse in research to evaluate the effectiveness of interventions where results are formulated and measured in terms of quality of life, quality adjusted life years, wellbeing and liveability. The wellbeing and satisfaction of the patient is therefore growing in prominence as a focus of policy and interventions. Earlier foci of concern on technical aspects of medicine – parodied in the adage 'the operation was a success but unfortunately the patient died' – have been supplemented by an emphasis on the subjective space of the patient as both an evaluative measure and a driver of policy.

The subjective wellbeing of the patient or client taking centre stage with their purported wants and needs providing the rationale for policy was apparent from the outset of the New Labour period. Early in New Labour's 1997–2010 time in office, this was underscored by a Cabinet Office document that wrote of 'making sure that public service users, not providers, are the focus' (Cabinet Office 1999, 6). The justification of the changes in the organization of health and welfare services that took place during this period of government drew upon several persuasive tropes which stressed change, efficiency, effectiveness, quality, choice and 'what the public actually want' (Scourfield 2007). The pursuit of change was presented as a necessary response to both a more demanding public and a fast changing world. The Cabinet Office paper went on to say:

> Too often in the past, the tendency in the public service has been to stick with the traditional. The world is changing too fast for that to be an effective approach. The best public bodies have shown an ability to innovate and improve. (Cabinet Office 1999, 35)

This document formulates the shifts in health and welfare policy in terms of responding to the 'needs of citizens and businesses', what matters to 'the people', 'what people really want' and changes that reflect 'real people's lives'. The principle of 'person centredness' was key to the proposed changes (Scourfield 2005).

Yet there is a tension in social and health policy in this period. The sovereignty of consumers of health and social care services and the power of their putative desires to determine policy are not untrammelled. The sovereignty of the individual citizen foregrounded in documents such as the Cabinet Office paper mentioned above is mitigated and sometimes directly undermined on a variety of other fronts. The way that the population responds to the new healthcare landscape is itself something that campaigners, managers and policymakers are keen to manipulate. From participation in screening programmes to exhortations to follow official advice, concerns with compliance with therapeutic regimes and the involvement of clients in planning and purchasing their own care, the sovereignty of the individual is itself a commodity that policymakers seek to colonize and shape.

In this chapter we will consider how a group of exemplary health initiatives have served to configure what it means to be an individual under advanced liberalism and how this yields novel forms of relationship between the individual and the state as well as new relationships between the citizen and his or her experiences of embodiment. As we shall suggest, these have on the one hand yielded an impetus towards greater responsibility on the part of individual citizens and on the other afforded means by which the state has become a key player in the relationship that we have with others, with ourselves and with our bodies.

Screening Ourselves to Health

Let us begin with the role of the medico-political complex in the relationship that citizens have with their bodies. Rather than being something immediately experienced – pains, pleasures, exuberance, fatigue and the like – our experience is increasingly expert mediated. Rather than rely on our own sense of the state of ourselves it is to tests, assays, investigations and screening that we turn to establish the state of ourselves and our health.

The expansion of screening programmes for disease has been one of the most remarkable features of the post–Second World War healthcare landscape in advanced liberal nations. Under contemporary medico-political regimes, the individual is hailed by a variety of initiatives to participate in screening activities ostensibly with a view to identifying early signs of disease and facilitating rapid, and therefore more, effective treatment. The individual is aided and shaped as a self-monitoring individual by means of such programmes, participation in which is urged by campaigners, central government and, increasingly, citizens themselves.

Screening programmes provide a particularly interesting case in point, because the effectiveness of some of these programmes in terms of making an actuarial difference to the morbidity and mortality of populations is somewhat debatable. Examples of programmes which afford minimal or even negligible protection in relation to the actuarial risk borne by the individual are easy to find in the medical literature. In the case of prostate cancer, a meta-analysis of several studies including nearly 400,000 participants by Djulbegovic, Beyth et al. (2010) concluded that there was no evidence that routine screening reduced mortality, yet it is still widely practiced and is mandatory under a number of health insurance schemes in the US. Cervical screening provides another example. Whilst widely practiced in many developed nations it is of limited value in reducing morbidity and mortality in younger women and only begins to detect practically significant rates of abnormality after the age of 34 (Sasieni, Castanon et al. 2009). Concerns are expressed about the alacrity with which younger women are embarked upon programmes of further investigation and treatment subsequent to detection of supposed abnormalities in cervical cells and the negative effects that treatment may have on their subsequent fertility (TOMBOLA Group 2009). Indeed, a 'more aggressive policy resulted in more overtreatment and adverse health events than the conservative option' (Franco 2009, 305).

Let us pursue the issue of cervical screening and cervical cancer as it illustrates some of the dynamics at the heart of the relationship between the state, medicine and the responsible individual. Whilst it is easy to find medical researchers and practicing doctors who are sceptical of the value of early screening (O'Mahony, Steedman et al. 2009), more popular accounts of the process display no such ambivalence. It is in this nexus that the popular media come to be crucial as communicators and formulators of issues. It is not that the media simply reflect the will of elite groups, nor do they necessarily shape public consciousness or reflect popular sentiments in any simple sense. Rather, it is because they are increasingly recognized as important policy actors in their own right (Baum and Potter 2008; Page 1996).

This imperative to screen was brought into particularly sharp focus by the extensively mass-mediated events surrounding the death of UK television personality Jade Goody (1981–2009), whose cervical cancer metastasized and resulted in her death. Her appearances in a number of so-called 'reality' television programmes in which participants spend a period of time in a closed environment devised by the programme makers, yielded a great deal of media coverage focusing especially on her behaviour on screen and her terminal illness. The detection of her rapidly metastasizing cancer with a tumour of the cervix resulted in coverage of her plight that activated a variety of debate about the condition and the desirability of screening.

Much was made of the 'Goody effect' or 'Jade's legacy', such that there was an increase in the uptake of cervical screening opportunities as a result of her death and associated publicity. This occasioned comment from politicians and journalists alike. An item from the *Daily Star* dated 23 October 2009 shows the process in action:

Health secretary Andy Burnham, 39, paid tribute to 'Jade's Legacy', which has seen the NHS test 12% more women aged 25–64 than it did last year. Charities and the Government said the increase, the first since 2002, was a result of the late TV star's brave fight against cancer. Mr Burnham said: 'These figures show the remarkable effect Jade's tragic case has had in reversing a downward trend in the number of young women attending cervical screening. Jade's bravery and openness in her fight against cervical cancer has brought home to young women across the country the importance of regularly going for these checks.'
(Pauley 2009, 13)

Certainly this highlights the political imperative to encourage more people through the screening process and thereby to manage their cervical cytology through the state-sanctioned medical complex. But it highlights considerably more than this. For one thing, it underscores the relationship between politics and celebrity such that politicians' public pronouncements are addressed to – and occasioned by – events in the world of celebrity rather than being guided by any independent political vision or popular mandate. In passing, we might note the use of the by now commonplace notion that those who succumb to cancer are 'brave', an adjective seldom applied to those who die of heart disease or hospital acquired infections. At the heart of this kind of reporting and embedded in the policy is the notion that our bodies are somehow dangerous if left unsupervised and that the management of these risks is best brought under the control of the medico-political complex. The relationship between the citizen and their own body is inherently suspect. Personal feelings of wellness or illness or the experience of symptoms which might prompt us to consult a doctor or retire to bed are insufficient to manage our bodies which have been freshly invested with risk. The job of responsible individuals is not to know themselves – for this information can be disclosed only by experts and laboratory procedures – but to responsibly participate in the process of investigation, measurement and control.

This is a process which is profoundly interior in a sense never achieved by the earlier welfarist programmes of inoculation, school milk and vitamin fortified orange juice in the decades immediately after the Second World War. The body is not to be trusted and is in need of professional supervision and expert vigilance. This new form of health and the corresponding novel forms of embodiment cannot be augmented simply by calorific intake or vaccination.

The desire of people themselves to bring their own bodies under such a regime is highlighted by the popular campaigns around the death of Jade Goody concerning the minimum age at which young women should commence being screened. The age at which invitations to report for screening are commenced is currently 25 years for women in England and 20 in Wales and Scotland. This discrepancy, allied to publicity surrounding Jade Goody's death, has occasioned a number of popular demands for the age to be lowered in England too despite limited evidence as to its benefits. The *Sun* promoted a campaign to lower the minimum screening age aided by a 'Jade's legacy' petition that was claimed to contain 178,000 signatures. The fact that this did not immediately lead to a change in government policy was met with chagrin voiced by the paper through the words of concerned readers who had supported the campaign. As one was reported to say:

> …the Government should hang their heads in shame for letting young women down. It is an outrage that after all the publicity over Jade's tragic, premature death and the other women who have bravely come forward to tell their stories, the Government still say women under 25 should not be tested. (*Sun* 2009, 42)

In this view the job, if not the purpose, of the state is to manage this relationship that individuals have with their bodies through the process of screening. The consumer citizen can therefore expect – and in some cases actively desire – to undergo this process. Indeed the evidence on which a decision not to screen ever younger women was derided:

> Tessa, of Croydon, Surrey, says: 'I'm gutted. The report seems to be all medical facts and figures. It's like they've taken no notice of our personal plights.' (*Sun* 2009, 43)

The actuarial risks and their likely reduction by more inclusive screening is here irrelevant to the desire of the citizen to avail herself of this procedure and for the government to address the 'plight' of those like herself who feel that they need a smear test. The situation of Jade Goody was highly atypical and involved a particularly rapid and aggressive disease affecting her colon, bladder and liver as well as her cervix. Yet in campaigns like this she was reformulated as the mundane sufferer from abnormalities, the cytological everywoman representing the potential fate of all those who are not screened early or often enough.

Jade Goody's posthumous lifesaving properties were underscored by further articles in the popular press. In March 2010, the *Sun* ran an item featuring the stories of women who had undergone cervical smear tests that had yielded evidence of abnormalities entitled 'We only had cancer test thanks to Jade... she saved our lives; Jade's Legacy one year on: The women she saved' (Wighton 2010). One of the women quoted in the article reportedly said:

> Every young woman who read Jade's story must have been moved and called to action to get tested, knowing it can strike any woman at any age. Like Jade, I also had two sons – Corey, who's now 13, and Dylon, who's ten – and the thought of leaving them motherless filled me with dread...
> In April I went to my GP for a test, waited six weeks for the results, then got the news that some abnormal cells had been detected. Further tests found cancer cells, graded at the lowest 1A1 level, so while it was bad news, at least they had caught it early. (Wighton 2010, 26)

This quotation shows how immediate the putative benefits are. A smear test will catch the process early before serious damage is done. Thus the prudent prophylactic aspects of testing are foregrounded as is the apparent near inevitability of discovering the need for further treatment. Following the trajectory of Jade Goody means that one's relationship with one's own body is mediated through celebrity as well as by the state and underscores the dangerousness of the reproductive tract especially in women. 'I won't let my girls wait until they're 25 before they have a smear test' opined Paul Carter, whose byline described him as a 'consultant gynaecologist' in the *Daily Mail* (Carter 2010). These are popular press reports rather than scientific documents or policy statements, but they are particularly revealing here because they illustrate how the segue is achieved between illness and the desirability of screening as if this were a seamless process.

Since its association with the human papillomavirus, cervical cancer has become a condition into which has been decanted a good deal of the unease about sexuality itself. It incorporates important tropes about the dangerousness of sex and its suitability for medical management that were thoroughly established in the nineteenth century. In this view, sexuality and reproductive health are not properly matters of self-management but instead are too hazardous to be entertained without expert supervision.

Screening places individuals in a state of enforced and extended infancy. Whilst the offspring mentioned in Carter's article might be thought to be able to make their own minds up in their 20s, decisions regarding screening are formulated as a matter of responsible parenthood, the reach of whose mission extends far beyond the legal age of majority. Liberated from any need to make an actuarial difference to a person's morbidity or risk, screening takes on a life of its own as a part of the relationship between the self and a larger polity, and as part of responsible self-management. Citizens themselves campaign for their right to be screened independently of actuarial evidence that it might make a difference to the health of the population as a whole in their particular age group. The subjective territory of the citizen has been sufficiently colonized by notions of risk, the hazardousness of our bodies and the practices of intimacy with others for this to make sense.

Cervical examination is not alone. There are many further examples of screening processes which proliferate even more independently of actuarial risk. In the case of breast cancer, mammograms have been widely deployed as a screening tool with a view to reducing the toll of mortality and morbidity from breast cancer. Schemes to enhance the uptake of these kinds of programmes are widely reported in the literature and projects to increase the availability and acceptability of screening programmes are commonplace, yet there is still considerable debate as to whether the burden of morbidity and mortality can be significantly altered as a result of such interventions. The US Preventive Services Task Force (2009) recommended a restriction in the age groups invited into screening programmes, pointing especially to the negligible benefits for those aged under 50 years or over 75. Indeed, the case for screening may be even less convincing, for as McPherson (2010, 341) points out, the pooled benefits from studies on participants aged under 60 years are of 'marginal statistical significance while some large trials show no benefit'. Some authors point to the significant risks of overdiagnosis – that is where lesions are detected that would not be life-threatening if they were left alone, yet involve the patient being strongly encouraged to embark on further investigations and treatment which themselves carry significant risks (Jørgensen and Gøtzsche 2009).

Despite this ambiguity about the value of such schemes in the scientific literature, there is considerable enthusiasm for them. The impulse toward certitude and surveillance remains a powerful guiding principle at the level of policy and healthcare practice. Moreover, health screening and the institutional management of risk involve an alliance of global capital – notably the biotechnology industry – as well as entrepreneurs and private investors providing services, clinicians and scientists from an array of disciplinary and national backgrounds, and politicians and social policy makers concerned to manage the growing cost of health and welfare provision. Allied to this is the conviction among many clinicians and providers of screening services that they are on the front line of saving lives, as revealed in letters to the *Annals of Internal Medicine* subsequent to the publication of the US Preventive Services Task Force report (US Preventive Services Task Force 2009).

Notions of individual choice and personal responsibility permeate these new clinical services as citizens are encouraged to participate in testing schemes as if this were the right and responsible thing to do. People whose results show them to be at risk of more serious or life-threatening conditions are treated as if their state is a temporary aberration. They are in what Bauman (1997) called a state of 'suspended extinction'. Their subsequent choices can then be moulded to reduce the likelihood of their incipient condition developing and the outcome of the courses of treatment to which they will be subject will result in their eventual reassimilation as 'normal, healthy' individuals.

The values of doubt, uncertainty, choice, individuality and risk which pervade reflexive modernity have not entirely supplanted older modernist values of objectivity, order, progress and certainty. The idea that screening will allow us to identify early stage disease before it becomes life-threatening is still a potent one. The imperative to impose orderliness on the human world inherent in screening programmes reflects the impetus of governmentality towards universal classification and normalization.

Screening also invites pre-modern notions of fatalism and destiny that are reconfigured in contemporary programmes such that it is the 'abnormal' cells, the antigens or the lesions visible via radiography that are deemed to foretell the individual's destiny. Unlike earlier metaphysical notions of destiny or nineteenth-century ideas of disease as a process of infection or contagion, here the location of the destiny is placed firmly within the individual. In addition, the medical warrant for the proposed origins of disease disclosed by testing shifts the emphasis from social provision or amelioration towards medical intervention with respect to a range of impairments, diseases and behaviours (Lippman 1991; Rose 1994).

Once risks of this kind have become medicalized, and the notion that screening is a desirable end in itself has been secured among many health campaigners and a proportion of the public and the political class, other possibilities are unfolded for the development of what Foucault (1988) and Rose (1996) would call governmentality. The process of medicalizing the risks inherent in the human body and the screening processes designed to ferret these out opens the possibility of new arrays of rules for the conduct of one's own everyday existence. The citizen's energy, initiative, ambition, calculation and personal responsibility should properly be directed towards detecting and managing these risks in themselves. Entrepreneurial individuals will make it part of the enterprise of their lives to maximize their own human capital, project themselves a future and seek to shape their lives in terms of these procedures which aim to detect and manage the risks involved, in order to become what they wish to be. Under this kind of regime, where the management of one's own health is foregrounded, the enterprising self is active and calculating so as to better itself in the topography of internal risk (Rose 1996, 154). In this sense, the autonomy of the citizen involves taking control of our undertakings, defining our goals and planning to achieve our needs through our own powers to participate in the rituals of health (Rose 1996, 159). Yet, where screening is concerned, the recommended process of calculation does not derive directly from the research literature or the debate this has fostered in medical journals. It is as if the imperative of screening itself should be taken for granted and the calculations undertaken by the individual should proceed from this point.

Screening Spaces: Technologies of Governmentality and Preventative Healthcare

The expansion of screening has brought with it a new academic focus on the reasons why people do not comply with screening programmes. For the most part, this literature sidesteps the question of whether such programmes confer any appreciable benefit to the individual as we have described above. One might suppose that there is at least room for debate and doubt among well informed individuals. The literature on screening uptake and adherence, however, is beset by no such uncertainty. Instead it takes the benefit of screening as if it were pre-given: 'Given the possible life-threatening health ramifications of not following established cancer screening recommendations, why do so many women fail to comply?' ask Goldenberg, Routledge et al. (2009, 563). Researchers have focused on the indigenous beliefs of immigrant groups as representing a barrier to screening (Chavez, Hubbell et al. 1995; Tejeda, Thompson et al. 2009), as if localized scepticism were somehow quaintly primitive and could be swept away with better education and publicity. A theatre of operations is opened up inside the potential participant's head, which can be manipulated by the astute health educator. The interior stage is populated with features and entities which may be rearranged, reduced or enhanced to increase the likelihood of a desired outcome. Possible complicating factors may include neuroticism or a form of existential dread caused by awareness of one's mortality that may get in the way of participation in screening programmes (Goldenberg, Routledge et al. 2009). The sphere of operations of the persuasive process can extend to the potential participant's immediate social circle too. The observation that participants in screening programmes have been persuaded by family members to report for screening has led to suggestions that relatives should be enlisted by programme promoters as an additional source of leverage on the citizen deemed to be in need of screening (Tejeda, Thompson et al. 2009).

Once screening test results are available, there is a variety of material and practical forces at work to place the individual deemed at risk on a kind of conveyor belt of further investigation and intervention. A number of material factors, such as limited consultation time, the urge from both clients and professionals for a decisive diagnosis, added to a medical desire to intervene if any abnormality is discovered often mean that suggestions of abnormality in screening results gain the status of definitive diagnoses. As well as the physical body, the interior subjective space becomes a site of intervention for clinicians and health educators with counselling and education being included as well as more physically invasive tests and interventions, prophylactic treatment and further monitoring and evaluation. Doubt or ambivalence is privatized (Bauman 1997) as individuals and healthcare providers translate complex and often ambivalent risk estimates into decisions about whether to proceed with further investigation or treatment, and meaningful life trajectories (Parsons and Atkinson 1992; Hallowell 1998).

Of course, individuals may elect not to be tested, be ambivalent about its benefits or merely forget to respond to the reminders, but the cultural and technological imperative remains such that despite the failure to lower the cervical screening age in England, the overall trend is for many policymakers and health educators to seek to make services more readily available, improve or reconfigure them so as to enhance their uptake. Many of the improvements suggested – such as using less subjectively intrusive techniques, making the socioemotional environment of the clinic more welcoming or improving communication – are resolutely fixed on individual or interpersonal issues rather than on the broader question of whether the practice does any good.

The experts urging us to participate in screening activities have accumulated to themselves a double authority. They have retained their power and resources to translate uncertainty into advice and information to health consumers. They have also acquired a corresponding moral authority, inasmuch as the course of action that they advocate is the right and proper responsible thing to do and to do otherwise represents some sort of deficiency on the part of the citizen. Notions of individual choice and responsibility are grounded in a discourse of certainty, scientific progress and success in the war against disease. Whereas, in the twentieth century, vaccination was the paradigmatic public health measure, in the twenty-first century screening has taken its place in developed nations. The alleged benefits and the often unmitigated desirability of screening pervades many professional and media accounts of the process. In best modernist style, the results of these procedures are constructed as if they were unproblematic facts about the human body such that its social context and the extent of its underlying actuarial support in the management of risk remain unexamined. Screening programmes and their associated publicity therefore continue to reflect modernist claims to ultimate knowledge about and control of human nature. It is a kind of knowledge that, despite its sometimes ambiguous scientific grounding, has a moral imperative attached to it as regards the responsible conduct of the citizen. Rather than being a matter of choice, responsibility itself is one of the factors urging compliance. The responsibilized citizen's realm of choice is circumscribed by some variant or other of education, expertise and subjection to allegedly rational processes of governance.

Compliance, Concordance and Adherence: Configuring the Responsible Patient

The question of adherence to screening regimes is one facet of a much larger area of concern in contemporary healthcare and health education. The question of whether responsible individuals in their role as patients actually follow the advice they are given has exercised healthcare practitioners, researchers and policymakers for some time. Once again, taking the wisdom of health advice or prescribed regimes of pharmacotherapy or conduct as if they were unproblematically desirable, the concern is whether patients do as they are told and how professionals might increase this likelihood. Patient compliance may be defined as 'the extent to which a person's behaviour cooperates with the medical suggestions he or she has been provided' (Kampman and Lehtinen 1990, 167). World Health Organization (WHO) estimates suggest that only 50 per cent of sufferers from long-term conditions pursue treatment as recommended by physicians (WHO 2003) and of prescriptions issued 20–30 per cent may not even be taken to a pharmacy (Fischer, Stedman et al. 2010).

From the point of view of practitioners and researchers, the 'problem' of patient non-compliance with recommended medical regimens has been extensively documented (Fincham 2007; Laude and Tabuteau 2007; Palazoolo and Olie 2004; Reach 2007). As Gueguen and Vion (2009, 689) stated:

This noncompliance is generally associated with wasted time for practitioners, a negative effect on patients' health, an increase in the number of relapses and, therefore, an increase in health-care costs.

Thus the aim is to educate, persuade and otherwise inform the patient of the likely costs to them, their loved ones and the healthcare system as a whole of their waywardness. There is an underlying assumption that non-compliance is to do with incompetence or incomplete knowledge on the part of the patient. Moreover:

> Non-adherence to treatments is also a major obstacle in translating efficacy in research settings into effectiveness in clinical practice. (Berk, Hallam et al. 2010, 2)

It is the patients' egregiousness then that prevents the treatment regime from working rather than, for example, exaggerated expectations about its effectiveness on the part of health professionals. Often it is proposed that this is because of some sort of deficiency or lack on the part of the patients. In the case of mental health conditions, Kao and Liu (2010, 557) say that in clinical settings many patients with schizophrenia appear to lack 'insight' into the 'illness' which often leads to therapeutic non-compliance. In Kao and Liu's own study, they found that 'patients with better medication compliance had better insight into mental illness, less severe psychopathologic condition, and less negative subjective response to side effects of antipsychotics'.

Notice how the apparently desirable quality of 'insight' is aligned with agreement with clinicians' views and the desirability of subscribing to a view of one's condition which posits medication as the most appropriate response. The side effects of antipsychotics, some of which are profoundly disabling, are well documented (Jacobs 1995; Reynolds and Kirk 2010; Seeman 2010). Consequently, the wisdom of 'compliance' is at least debatable. Nevertheless, the possibility that there may be different views on the desirability of medically sanctioned courses of action is generally not explored in the literature on compliance. Indeed, minimizing side effects on the part of the patient is as desirable inasmuch as it is associated with greater compliance, it seems.

In the health practice and health education communities there are some signs of disquiet with the notion of compliance. Attempts have been made to supplant this older physician-led approach with concepts that instead stress shared decision making and accord between the parties in the healthcare encounter. There is a growing preference for ideas such as 'adherence' and 'concordance' instead. These latter ideas it is said connote greater patient and carer involvement and agreement. For example:

> Adherence is defined as the extent to which health behaviour reflects a health plan constructed and agreed to by the patient as a partner with a clinician in health care decision making. (Gould and Mitty 2010, 290)

This relationship between the clinician and patient and the emphasis on mutual planning is itself advocated as a kind of therapeutic technology to bring patients into line with the wisdom of clinicians. This is often the underlying theme when researchers and clinicians talk of a 'therapeutic alliance'. Strauss and Johnson (2006) describe how a strong therapeutic alliance had a 'positive influence' on beliefs and attitudes so that clients appeared to have less negative attitudes about their medication, greater acceptance of doctor-approved views of their illness and improved adherence. In a similar vein, an earlier paper by Lingam and Scott (2002) also stressed the importance of therapeutic alliances indicating that non-adherence was four times more likely when clinician–patient interaction was reported to be poor.

The idea that relationships and interactions with health professionals themselves are tools for enabling greater likelihood of adherence or compliance has been behind a number of initiatives to promote discussions of medication use between patients and professionals in healthcare. Let us examine this in more detail via an examination of one UK initiative to promote this kind of consultation, the 'medication review'.

The process of medication review has been initiated recently in the UK, ostensibly so as (1) to increase compliance to prescribed medication regimes through the improvement of patients' knowledge and use of their drugs and (2) to reduce waste through improved clinical and cost effectiveness. The focus therefore is on gaining and improving compliance (NHS 2004, 2005). Key to this process are pharmacists who can visit clients in their own homes and discuss with them the medication and ensure that it is being taken as directed as well as to examine the possibility that prescribed medication may be interacting with any over-the-counter medicines which clients may be taking. Salter (2010) reported on a study of interactions between pharmacists and elderly clients. Rather than exemplifying the much-vaunted notions of concordance and adherence, it was clear that the pharmacists led the interview as if it were a kind of interrogation. The critical point of most of the medication reviews was whether the medication was being taken as directed, and Salter found little evidence of the two way processes envisaged in models of patient centred care or concordance. Like a number of other studies of pharmacist–patient interaction (Norris and Rowsell 2003; Skoglund, Isacson et al. 2003; Morrow, Hargie et al. 1993), Salter's work suggested that pharmacists have a tendency to adopt a protocol driven discourse involving eliminative questioning that can be technical, perfunctory and impersonal.

Medication review, rather than ensuring a participatory process of concordance between healthcare practitioners and clients, appeared to be firmly embedded within a public health paradigm which viewed non-compliance as due to ignorance, incompetence or poor patient understanding and any lapses require scrutiny and instruction from a healthcare professional. In Salter's study participants had gained little knowledge as a result of the medication review but instead – and perhaps more significantly from our point of view – they had been subject to the gaze of authority. Being elderly and having recently come out of hospital they were at pains to show that they were coping and were keen to deflect perceived threats to their autonomy.

In this way, we can see how a system of care that has ostensibly been set up to assist patients with medication issues and enhance safety serves as a disciplinary device to enforce compliance and to propel patients into a sometimes desperate display of autonomy and responsibility, apparently in an effort to deflect any possible suggestion that they are not coping. In this sense, even care itself can incite individuals to go to great lengths to show that they are autonomous and responsible.

Rather than developing a space of mutual agreement and shared planning in an equitable fashion between professionals and patients, it is possible (perhaps even likely) that consultations can function as further mechanisms to enforce compliance and impose a medically sanctioned agenda. The equality and agreement implied when compliance is refashioned into adherence or concordance may be more apparent than real. Indeed, it may make the possibility of resistance more remote.

The idea that an individual's personal or mental qualities may be crucial in their response to healthcare suggestions has been attracting the attention of a growing number of scholars. This new field which has been termed by its enthusiasts 'cognitive epidemiology' (Deary and Batty 2007), has attracted growing attention. In this instance, the determinants of health are reformulated and cognitive capacities are positioned as key determinants of health. As in *The Bell Curve* (Herrnstein and Murray 1994), inequalities are seen as stemming from differences in intelligence. Rather than, for example, socioeconomic status being seen as a key variable in the likelihood of mortality or morbidity, instead the mental qualities that correspond to this are proposed to underlie the observed differences. As Deary and Batty (2007, 378) say:

Since the start of the new millennium…low intelligence test scores have begun to appear in epidemiological reports as a risk factor for total mortality and possibly some disease specific outcomes, including coronary heart disease.

Thus, cognitive epidemiology reinstates and offers a scientific rationale to the idea of deficits in health representing some sort of intellectual deficit on the part of sufferers. Lubinski (2009) in an editorial in the journal *Intelligence*, consolidates this idea of a deficit in understanding and foresight as being responsible for the poorer health of the poorer members of advanced societies. A key facet of cognitive epidemiology, he says,

> addresses the judgment and decision-making required for developing a healthy lifestyle, avoiding health risks, and exercising preventive medicine. All of these tasks require cognitive competencies for acquiring and effectively using new information, which are of critical importance in modern societies, where people have the complex task of managing their own health care. (Lubinski 2009, 626)

An example of this kind of work can be seen in a study by Deary, Gale et al. (2009), who examined the relationship between verbal intelligence and persistence with a medication regime over two years among nearly 2000 people in Scotland. Those who scored highest on a measure called the Mill Hill Vocabulary Scale were most likely to persist with the medication. As Deary, Gale et al. (2009, 607) say:

> Such persisting with potentially helpful health behaviours in the face of uncertainty might partly explain why people with higher intelligence live longer and suffer less morbidity from chronic diseases.

Rather than the earlier socioeconomic concerns in epidemiology, this new trend is concerned with the interior landscape of the patient as a determining factor in their health. The responsible patient is also healthier, and this is determined by their greater intelligence. The more intelligent a person is, the more likely they are to make life decisions in line with recommendations and advice from health educators and professionals and the longer they live. The more compromised a person is according to the yardstick of reason, the poorer will be their health.

The ideas behind cognitive epidemiology share several commonalities with the ideas embedded in contemporary healthcare policy. It is the internal architecture of responsibility to which many policy initiatives are addressed, as we have seen, and the locus of risk is where possible devolved to the individual. But policy often goes further than this. The process of responsibilization not only accords with the idea that people who do not have a certain kind of mental architecture are disenfranchizing themselves from health and hence from society, but it actively tries to encourage the requisite structures and interior processes. Our next example will attempt to show this in action. The entrepreneurial citizen in neoliberal healthcare regimes is possessed of certain mental capacities – grasping the importance of taking responsibility for their health. The policy process can go to considerable lengths to try to install these capacities and in doing so using a great many concepts which appear to enhance the autonomy and emancipation of the individual.

Individual Budgets: The Devolution of Health and Social Care to the Individual

In this section, we will consider how the idea of an autonomous independent service user and the notion of an entrepreneurial citizen has been amalgamated with some of the more apparently radical rhetoric of service users movements from the 1960s and 1970s to afford a particular process of responsibilization for people with long-term health problems and disabilities. In the UK the manifest position of government policy is to promote service user choice and personalization in the provision of health and social care services. Where the care of people with persistent health problems or disabilities is concerned, a key document in this respect was the 2005 green paper 'Independence, Wellbeing and Choice' (Department of Health 2005) promising that:

> ...we want to provide better information and signposting to allow people to retain responsibility, and to put people at the centre of assessing their own needs and how those needs can best be met. (Department of Health 2005, 10)

This has proceeded in tandem with a personalization agenda that seeks to tailor services to particular individual circumstances such that 'every person across the spectrum of need' would have 'choice and control over the shape of his or her support, in the most appropriate setting' (Department of Health 2008, 2). This, claimed the New Labour government, would yield a desirable situation where

> people are able to live their own lives as they wish, confident that services are of high quality, are safe and promote their own individual requirements for independence, well-being and dignity. (Department of Health 2008, 2)

This was to be achieved by allocating people in need budgets of their own and placing them in the position of purchasers who would have considerable discretion in terms of the services they commissioned for themselves and who they bought them from:

> Over time, people who use social care services and their families will increasingly shape and commission their own services. Personal Budgets

will ensure people receiving public funding use available resources to choose their own support services. (Her Majesty's Government 2007, 2)

In line with this, a policy objective throughout the last two decades in the UK has been to promote a personalized model of adult social care that foregrounds choice and personalized support for disabled people and other service users.

It is not our intention to review the operation of personalized or individual budget schemes in their entirety. There is already a great deal of discussion of this elsewhere (Glasby, Le Grand et al. 2009; Glasby and Littlechild 2009; Individual Budgets Evaluation Network 2008). Rather, it is our intention to draw out some of the dilemmas of this means of funding and supporting care, and the implications for the process of responsibilization that we have identified.

As Rabiee and Moran (2006) indicate, the approach of individual budgets and their precursors has by now a long history. It builds on the experience of 'direct payments' for people with disabilities in the 1990s and the model of 'in control' developed with people with learning difficulties in the early twenty-first century. In the later part of the decade, 'individual budgets' were piloted with the manifest aim of enhancing users' choice and control. This approach means that individual service users are rather like businesses. They are provided with a budget and may commission services from relevant bodies and individuals both public and private. The rationales for 'direct payments', 'in control', 'personal budgets' (England) and 'individual budgets' (Scotland) all drew upon the notion of person-centred planning (Dowling, Manthorpe et al. 2006) and individualization and represent an approach to welfare that substitutes 'cash' for centrally provided 'care' in some areas of provision (Glendinning and Kemp 2006; Ungerson and Yeandle 2007). Overall, a recent evaluation of the scheme (Hatton and Waters 2011) suggests a degree of satisfaction with it among users and carers, and widespread uptake with around a third of those eligible for local authority funded care in England receiving some sort of direct payment or personal budget (Jerome 2011). This change in the way that welfare is administered to people with disabilities is mooted to represent a major shift in the paradigm of the relationship between the citizen and the state. This new model, say Henwood and Hudson (2008, 9), involves three concepts, namely user control, choice of service and flexibility of support.

The degree of autonomy granted to people with disabilities making use of these schemes and the kinds of service and activities on which the money was spent has led to some intriguing proliferation of debate. In particular, press reports of personal budget schemes have tended to draw upon a rich seam of ambivalence about the relationship of people with disabilities to pleasure, leisure and sexuality. The direct payments scheme was subject to a surge of media interest in August 2010 when the *Sunday Telegraph* reported that disabled people had used their personal budgets to pay for services from sex workers, visits to lap dancing clubs, internet dating services and holidays (Donnelly, Howie et al. 2010). The *Telegraph* reported that a selection of councils contacted had defended their position in terms of the activities funded contributing to the personal and/or mental wellbeing of the claimants, and if they were legal, stressing the degree of autonomy afforded by the budget scheme and the discretion granted to the claimant. The vast majority of authorities contacted said they did not have a policy on the topic and some of the examples quoted bore a striking resemblance to those in the Individual Budgets Evaluation Network (2008) report and the *How to be in control* DVD (In Control 2006); thus the degree of novelty in the news stories was somewhat debatable. What is intriguing here is the intersection of concerns about disability and sexuality. The *Daily Mail* (Sims 2010) reported that '53 per cent of the councils were said to have a strategy that "explicitly empowered" disabled people to pursue their sexual aspirations', which, whilst it did not specifically mention paid-for sexual encounters, enabled a slippage between the notion of 'sexual aspirations' and commercial sex. The subsequent debate elicited a sympathetic response from many quarters, as a variety of commentators, organizations and disabled people made the point that there was no reason why disabled people should not be sexually active if that activity was legal. In the *Daily Mail* article quoted above, a social worker was reported as saying that one of the claimants involved, 'a man of 21 with learning disabilities…has been to two sexual health and sexual awareness courses and basically wants to try it… Wouldn't you prefer that we can control this, guide him, educate him, support him to understand the process and ultimately end up satisfying his needs in a secure, licensed place where his happiness and growth as a person is the most important thing?' (Sims 2010). This quote appeared to be repeating statements made in a discussion forum[1] several months earlier which whilst reducing the apparent originality of the news article indicates the generality of these concerns. The issue of the sex lives of disabled people remains problematic (Kim 2011), having been subject to a surge of interest in the 1990s (*inter alia*, Shakespeare, Gillespie-Sells et al. 1996; O'Toole and Bregante 1992). As well as foregrounding rights on the part of people with disabilities, this debate imbued their 'needs' with a primordial, fundamental quality – 'basic drives, or the desire for love, affection and intimacy' (Milligan and Neufeldt 2001, 92). This has opened up for discussion in the public sphere as well as in the academic and practitioner

---

1 See http://www.communitycare.co.uk/carespace/forums/sex-and-social-work-this-thread-isnt-as-filthy-6999.aspx (accessed 7 December 2011).

literature a space in which the sexualities of people with disabilities can be discussed.

Returning to the example above, the language of the 'social worker' quoted (and other contributors to the online discussion board at Community Care) draws heavily on the language of control and the production of the docile citizen. The fuzzy notion of personal growth is mentioned, yet the rest of the quote suggests that this young man's sexuality had, in an important sense, been nurtured and controlled by 'experts'. This impression is sustained through examination of more academic literature. Kazukauskas and Lam (2009, 16) discuss the centrality of sexuality to rehabilitation, writing about it as a 'competency' underscoring the tutelary, pedagogic quality of contemporary incarnations of sex for clients and rehabilitation counsellors.

The question of whether the newly responsibilized recipients of payments and personal budgets are spending responsibly and what kinds of expenditure social services departments and carers should permit, illustrates one of the key recent shifts in the kind of person the disabled individual is imputed to be. As it has been styled by some commentators, the 'cash for care' model is deemed to be unlike any previous models of integrated care or interagency collaboration, the notion of individual budgets placing the individual service user as the driver of change in services. In doing this, as Scourfield (2007) argued, New Labour performed a deft political manoeuvre in bringing together the emancipatory aspirations of the disability movement and a neoliberal vision of an enterprise society. The cash for care recipient is, in this view, not a passive recipient of benefits but instead an enterprising entrepreneur and a self-sufficient manager who takes on responsibilities previously assumed by the public services themselves, and to make judgements about the prudent disposal of his or her budget – judgements which, as we have seen, may be contested by journalists and other policy actors. This apparently radical agenda is not only aligned with the neoliberal enterprise of responsibilization but is also aligned with a desire to cut costs as fiscal containment has been a significant propeller for a cash for care agenda in England, Wales and beyond (Yeandle and Ungerson 2007). When the *Sunday Telegraph* reported that a man with psychiatric problems received personal budget funding 'on top of his state benefits' to pay for a holiday in Tunisia with a friend, it was noted by the man himself that the holiday was cheaper than a week in institutional care (Donnelly, Howie et al. 2010).

The care workforce employed by these new entrepreneurs was likely to be cheaper, less skilled and considerably more casualized than any employed by healthcare organizations or social services departments. It is therefore also more likely to be 'grey labour' (James 2008), with few protections under employment law. This kind of arrangement is likely to be encouraged because

the budgets and payments to individual clients are likely to be set at a lower
value than the cost of equivalent care from a statutory provider (James 2008).
There is also a possibility that those who have been allocated a budget will
have to rely in large part upon informal family caregivers. Rabiee and Moran
(2006, 13) noted that:

> The common perception among these carers was that the families were
> expected to provide a high level of support on an informal basis and
> unpaid basis but that this contribution was not recognized.

The implementation of individual budget schemes therefore responsibilizes not
only clients, but also caregivers. There is an additional administrative burden,
including managing the paperwork for the budget and recruiting personal
assistants, that was identified in the government's own evaluation of the pilot
scheme (Individual Budgets Evaluation Network 2008). The concerns on the
part of clients included what would happen if they overspent or if they filled
in a form wrongly and the difficulty in recruiting suitable carers. Those who
were easily able to manage the additional responsibilities tended to be those
with personal and familial resources on which they could draw, for example
if they had previously served as a treasurer for an organization or if a relative
was an accountant.

   In this way a good deal of the burden of responsibility is devolved to the
individual recipient. This does not necessarily mean that the statutory agencies
are correspondingly relieved for they often have to maintain personnel to
work in parallel with this devolution of responsibility. In the name of making
services more personalized, the responsibilities upon the recipient of care
and their carers have multiplied. A community psychiatric nurse related an
interesting anecdote to us. She had had been employed in the same region
of Wales for over two decades and had known many of her clients from the
1980s as they entered and left the large residential hospital that had previously
served the region, then as they attended the day centre that she managed in
the 1990s with the move to 'community care'. In the final year of her career
before her recent retirement, one major part of this nurse's role had been to
run self-confidence classes for the service users to enable them to interview
people for positions as their own carers. The nurse told us that for many of
her patients in receipt of individual budgets a major concern had been the
prospect of holding such interviews – some of these patients had never been
interviewed for a job themselves, let alone interviewed anyone else. As other
commentators have noted, this places the client of personal budget schemes
as a recipient of information, education and advice from health professionals
and budget advisors as to how and on whom the money most prudently might

be spent (Baxter and Glendinning 2011) thus emphasizing even further the tutelary process of constructing the enterprising disabled citizen.

A feature of interest in this process of responsibilization is the way that it appropriates the once radical rhetorics of personal freedom, user involvement and user choice to vouchsafe this manoeuvre. As a number of authors including Carey (2009) and Jones (2005, 41–80) highlight, the hegemonic form of governance under neoliberalism is able to deploy discourse in a particularly supple and agile manner so as to appear to compromise and unite with what were once counter-hegemonic forces. In the case of healthcare, the proliferation of rhetoric foregrounding the supposed needs and preferences of service users and carers shows how the language of these groups has been adopted and their interests appropriated, which may actually serve to assimilate and quash many formerly emancipatory and counter-hegemonic tendencies in service user movements. Carey (2009) notes that the state's tendency to adopt counter-hegemonies and utilize them for very different purposes has been pivotal in relation to concepts such as social exclusion, empowerment and service user participation. Hegemonic forms of governance have been able to exploit ambiguities in formerly emancipatory concepts, dynamics, movements and philosophies and transform them into technologies of government rather than means of liberation. As Carey (2009, 182) reminds us, one of the features of a free market and neoliberal philosophy is its capacity to accommodate diffuse agendas, especially those that seek to claim and extend greater freedoms for all. As a response to the outcry from NHS managers, trades unions and professional bodies representing NHS workers, patients groups, charities, the media and many politicians in the wake of the UK coalition government's Health and Social Care Bill, itself proposing very neoliberal reforms to the NHS in England, in one speech David Cameron commented that these reforms would, among all the many other benefits, 'empower service users'.

Conclusion

The process of responsibilization in health proceeds across a variety of fronts. In many instances across the field of health and social care, the ideal individual is conceptualized as one who manages their health or their role as a discerning and prudent consumer of services, but there is much more than this. As we have shown with the debates and media coverage surrounding screening processes, these have in significant ways successfully been disarticulated from measured statistical risk. The operation of these as public phenomena is, in many important ways, concerned with the reconfiguration of selfhood as much as it is with any reduction in morbidity and mortality. The extent to which individuals can be hailed and inducted by these kinds of schemes and inveigled into participating is formulated in terms of their internal psychic architecture. Under these policy and health education imperatives, it is minds that must be regulated as much as potential bodily pathologies and the interior architecture reconfigured to render individuals more concordant with advice. In some circles at least, epidemiology is coming to be seen as a matter of intelligence rather than older welfarist constructs of poverty, socioeconomic differentials or gradients of access to services. So pervasive is the entrepreneurial imperative that even those who are longer term service users with severe and enduring disabilities are hailed by welfare systems that attempt to enfranchise them as managers of their own budgets. Whilst this might confer greater flexibility in the services acquired, it also forms an important means of engendering an enterprising frame of mind and consolidating the responsibilization process. Yet this process does not necessarily proceed evenly or smoothly. The possibility of clients spending their money on things that might be considered frivolous, or morally or politically inopportune evinces lines of fracture and dissent. The citizen's entrepreneurial autonomy as a consumer, a manager of their own care services or as a sexual citizen is nurtured, advised and managed by a variety of others, from relatives, carers and social workers through to the organs of the press as policy actors in their own right. The question of health illustrates particularly graphically how there is an oscillation between the poles of autonomy on the one hand and supplicatory compliance on the other.

Chapter Five

MENTAL HEALTH AND PERSONAL RESPONSIBILITY

Introduction: Responsibilizing Distress

Personal responsibility is urged upon clients of the mental health services as never before. From informal conversations between clients and professionals to national policy documents, the collective mindset has been configured so that responsibility is extolled as a means to rehabilitation and a therapeutic outcome in its own right (Newnes and Radcliffe 2005). This might seem like a rather grand statement on its own. It may seem to differ little from the conventional advice to the downhearted to 'pull yourself together' and it might seem unsurprising that professional intervention imbibes something of this cultural commonplace.

Yet the presence of discourses of responsibility in the field of mental health discloses some curious tensions and contradictions. The first and perhaps the most obvious of these is that it coexists with a competing tendency in mental health research and practice, which is to see the person as primarily a biological being, propelled by genetic predispositions, neurological organization and the ebb and flow of neurotransmitters and accompanying medications. Popular science, pharmaceutical advertising and many researchers in the field themselves encourage us to see ourselves in these terms – it is as if matters of biography and milieu have been 'molecularised' (Niewhoner 2011). There is a palpable enthusiasm for psychiatric genomics and this has become firmly embedded within systems of psychiatric research (Baart 2010) despite the ambitious overinterpretation of what are often tentative, ambiguous or negative findings (Crow 2008). For commentators such as Abraham (2010), there has been a significant growth in the tendency to see many aspects of health and disease in pharmaceutical terms, such that failures and deviations of our bodies and minds can be addressed through the use of pharmaceuticals. The biological sciences thus emerge as significant new actors upon the social stage, continuing but also extending their history of engagement with the human and policy disciplines (Rose 2007). On the face of it, this might mitigate against strong attributions of responsibility. If aspects of conduct are seen as manifestations of an underlying and causally prior biology, this might squeeze the conceptual domain in which responsibility might be exercised. Instead, as we shall see, the present day biologization of the human condition has afforded new spaces for the emergence of responsibility and attributions of culpability on the part of patients or clients. The very determinism attached to many contemporary understandings of mental ill health has fostered not a spirit of therapeutic optimism, but rather a sense of therapeutic hopelessness on the part of clinicians.

A further point of note in the domain of debate in the field of mental health is the sheer pervasiveness of so-called mental disorder. From the US National Comorbidity Survey (Kessler, Berglund et al. 2005) it appeared that around half the US population had experienced a mental disorder at some time in their lives. In Europe, a recent review of existing epidemiological studies, sample surveys and other data sets suggested that every year over a third of the European population suffers from mental disorders (Wittchen, Jacobi et al. 2011). In a sense, mental ill health has been democratized such that it has the potential to be the concern of every man or woman rather than a minority interest. The ongoing development of category systems, such as the forthcoming fifth edition of the American Psychiatric Association's *Diagnostic and Statistical Manual* (DSM), takes place against the background of a growing inclusion of the population in one or more diagnostic categories. Verhoeff (2010) and Wittchen, Jacobi et al. (2010) estimate that mental ill health or, as they prefer to call it, 'brain disorders', account for around 27 per cent of the burden of morbidity on the European population. The extent to which, under present-day regimes of epidemiological research, that we can be viewed as suffering from a mental disorder means that negotiating questions of responsibility is of considerable importance. Rather than merely addressing a special subset of the population, i.e., those who are ill, health professionals and particularly mental health professionals, have a potentially much wider remit. Where the disorder ends and personal volition begins, how one might responsibly conduct oneself in the face of a mental disorder and the relative role of social support networks, primary care, specialist mental health services and even the criminal justice system, are all up for grabs.

In tandem with this growing pervasiveness of knowledge about mental ill health and the growing tendency to see sufferers from mental ill health as what Rose has called 'somatic individuals' (Novas and Rose 2000), it is possible to see also the tendency of responsibilizing individuals in terms of mental health and illness itself. The failure to 'take responsibility' may be seen as one of a variety of conditions that Marina Valverde (1999) has termed 'diseases of the will', with a concomitant inference that the failure of responsibility has a causal basis in individual constitutional factors. Seeing a failure of responsibility in the patient, client or citizen as pathology paves the way toward some important mutations in how we think about and act upon the world and provides new ways in which clients of public services and mental health patients specifically are exhorted to act upon themselves.

In mental healthcare, an important milestone in the present era of active citizenship was marked by the publication of the UK 'National Service Framework for Mental Health' (Department of Health 1999) and where there has been a renewed emphasis on user consultation and participation. Yet increased user participation brings with it an emphasis on responsibility (Elstad and Eide 2009), both on the part of managers and practitioners whose job it is to solicit user participation, and upon the users who are under this approach encouraged to take the role of experts on their conditions, their care and its delivery.

To add to the complexity, the UK's system of administering services and benefits is undergoing a period of change. With the implementation of new policies from the coalition government starting in 2010, the system of benefits previously available to citizens with long-term illnesses and disabilities, including mental health problems, is in the process of restriction and retraction. People on Incapacity Benefit are to be migrated to a new benefit called Employment and Support Allowance, and in the process are scheduled to undergo a work capability assessment. Initiated in 2008, Employment and Support Allowance was intended to replace Incapacity Benefit and involves a strong focus on work capability assessment and work focused interviews as a condition of its being paid. The government's ambition is to transfer around a quarter of Incapacity Benefit claimants onto Employment and Support Allowance with the consequent obligation to seek work, and represents a retrenchment aimed at managing the demands that incapacitated individuals can make upon the public purse (Grover and Piggott 2010). The work capability assessment for Employment Support Allowance is more stringent than the personal capability assessment for the benefit this is replacing (Roxburgh 2011). Yet this is not the end of the story. Further reforms are planned, such that a range of benefits including Employment and Support Allowance will be replaced by a scheme termed Universal Credit (Department for Work and Pensions 2010).

Thus it is possible to detect an emphasis on refashioning the incapacitated citizen, including those with a variety of mental health problems, so as to be able to participate once more in the workforce. The focus of concern and intervention is the individual (who is mandated and incentivized) rather than, for example, addressing the labour market itself or the possibility of exclusionary practices in employment. Embedded in this is a particular model of work and economic activity that involves the individual going to work for a larger organization and receiving wages. As economies transform themselves and diversify, this is clearly not the only form of economic activity available, yet the impaired individual is seen as someone who should be readying themselves in terms of employability skills and movement towards enhanced 'independence'.

The degree to which this is a relatively recent sociopolitical accomplishment can be gauged by the fact that in the UK the custom and practice of mental healthcare has shifted in the past generation. Once, patients could live out their entire lives in hospital and there are frequent mentions of cases where a teenage pregnancy in the early twentieth century could lead to a lifetime in institutions. In describing the hospitalization of women who were judged to be 'mentally defective', Hilliard (1954, 1373) says that 'illegitimate pregnancy was the precipitating factor in the majority of cases'. By contrast, nowadays the impetus is towards rehabilitation and reintegration into all too often inhospitable communities and workplaces. Clients are propelled by a variety of health and social care professionals towards rehabilitative programmes, courses of education and employment itself, in the belief that this will benefit them and relieve the burden on an overstretched public purse.

This shift is pushing forward on a variety of fronts. There is legislation, such as the Disability Discrimination Act (1995) which has so far met with limited success in enhancing the employment prospects of people with mental health difficulties (Biggs, Hovey et al. 2010). There are, as we have discussed briefly above, changes in the kinds and availability of benefits upon which the incapacitated citizen might draw. As some commentators have noted in the popular press, there has been a resurgence of discourse on welfare benefits and their claimants, emphasizing the notion that they are 'workshy', 'cheats' and 'scroungers' (Garthwaite 2011), thus underscoring the putatively voluntary nature of long-term incapacity and sequestration from the labour force.

In tandem with these ideological manoeuvres, in our own research on the healthcare systems of England and Wales we have witnessed clients who fail to make progress being said to 'not really want to get better', or who are believed not to be complying with medication regimes on purpose so as to prolong their illness. The assumption that clients should be able to make progress and pull themselves up by their bootstraps in the face of severe disabilities or incapacitating side effects of treatment is apparently becoming more fashionable and is aligned with the powerful amalgam of culpability and mental distress as a failure of the will. Yet Burrows and Greenwell (2007, 4), in a refreshingly candid review of mental health services in Wales, went as far as to comment that 'service users continue to routinely encounter professional behaviour and attitudes that inhibit recovery'.

That is the manifest position vis-à-vis recovery and employment. Clients of health, social care and state benefits systems are assisted back into employment through various fiscal and bureaucratic processes. Yet looking at the broad sweep of policy and service implementation, it is possible to detect lines of fracture. In contrast to the apparently smooth conveyor belt that will propel distressed and incapacitated clients back to work, especially where those with mental health problems are concerned, there is a growing body of evidence to suggest that dedicated services for their problems are becoming more difficult to access. Burrows and Greenwell (2007, 4) noted that 'Good services are developed by serendipity rather than by design. This leaves many people in a public system of chance, hoping, rather than believing, that their needs will be met'. This picture is sustained elsewhere in the UK, where access to care is investigated (Audit Scotland 2009; Samele, Seymour et al. 2006). Even people who might be considered resourceful in accessing care, such as doctors themselves, have encountered difficulty (Stanton and Randall 2011). The responsibility discourse has coincided with a retraction in services in many nations (Elstad and Eide 2009), which in the UK has only partly been effected by statutory means. In part at least, the sheer difficulty of accessing benefits and services represents a sort of de facto management of demand for services.

In recent years, the UK has seen a huge number of failures and tragedies in the care of people with mental health problems, and many such cases have found their way into the media if they have involved violence or death. Whilst the sheer volume of these cases, the associated press coverage, inquiries and reports means that a comprehensive survey is beyond the scope of this chapter, we shall draw on a number of these events by way of illustration. Once again, our purpose is not to take these as being literally true in any simple sense, but in acknowledgement of the role of the press as policy actors and as an indicator of the kinds of discourses around responsibility and the apportionment of culpability which may be deployed. A number of these accounts are noteworthy for the degree to which they illustrate the attribution of responsibility to the individual concerned and the associated retreat of service providers from the case in the run-up to the tragedy.

The press in the UK – particularly local newspapers – often report cases where people with mental health problems and their carers describe obstructive and dismissive treatment, resonating with the more sober accounts of such difficulty from audit bodies and charitable organizations. In 2010 in Camarthen, a local paper reported the complaints of the mother of a client of the local mental health services as follows: 'Jamie Thomas Mosey, had begged unsuccessfully to be sectioned just hours before he hung himself. Jamie was labeled "attention seeking" and told to "get a job" by mental health workers, Mrs Mosey said. Just hours later, on June 9, he was dead' (Smith 2010, 31).

This is particularly germane to our argument here, typifying the trend noted by Burrows and Greenwell (2007), Audit Scotland (2009) and Samele, Seymour et al. (2006). Getting access to support is often hard work in itself and requests for service are seen as part of the problem – 'attention seeking'. The curative power of employment is urged upon distressed and confused citizens as if it were a panacea. How hard-pressed managers and workmates in the commercial sector are supposed to cope with the afflicted person's symptoms when trained professionals are unwilling to do so is uncertain in the light of the demonstrable difficulties in obtaining and sustaining employment experienced by people with mental health problems (Goldberg 2005; Perkins and Rinaldi 2002; Thornicroft 2006). Yet the message, from quotes attributed to practitioners in the local press to the broader shifts in legislation and benefit eligibility criteria, is that the workplace is where these dramas should be played out rather than the clinic.

As an alternative to the workplace, another major site of action for the management of those with mental health problems is the courtroom and ultimately the prison. In 2004, investigative journalist Nick Davies claimed that around 70 per cent of people in prison had mental health problems (Davies 2004). Later in the decade the All-Party Parliamentary Group on Prison Health (2006) quoted figures to the effect that 90 per cent of people in prison suffered from mental health problems with many of these having two or more, a figure repeated in the Bradley Report (2009). This includes those who enter prison with drug problems, who are believed to account for about half of all prisoners. Whilst many workers in the field and influential academic contributors to policy agree that this is not a desirable state, a great many people with mental health problems have continued to find their way into prison (Appleby, May et al. 2010). Aside from prison itself, there are a variety of 'disposal options' which involve restrictions and court mandated stipulations in the community. There are numerous reports of Anti-Social Behaviour Orders (ASBOs) being awarded against people whose behaviour suggested distress or mental health difficulty. Such cases include the ASBO awarded against a woman banning her from jumping into rivers or canals after she repeatedly threw herself into the River Avon, or the ASBO granted against a man with mental health problems preventing him from sniffing petrol at petrol stations (Urquhart 2009). The deployment of ASBOs reflects what some commentators have seen as an emphasis on enforcement under New Labour (Hodgkinson and Tilley 2011) and as MacDonald (2006) notes, ASBOs are activated as a form of social control where a variety of social difficulties indicative of mental health problems are concerned, which often accelerates the individual on a path towards custodial sanction.

On a number of fronts, from benefit and employment policies to a variety of processes which subject those with mental health problems to criminal or

civil sanction, the UK's policies in mental healthcare are becoming imb
with the notion that clients and their carers should 'take responsibility' for their
actions rather than merely be cared for. Exhorting clients toward responsibility
is aligned with the broader notions of responsible citizenship described earlier,
with the tendencies described by critical scholars as 'neoliberal penality'
(Harcourt 2010). The tendencies in psychiatry, neuroscience, pharmaceutical
advertising and behaviour genetics to see the individual as propelled by
determinate and determining forces coexist, as Rose (2010) notes, with a
tendency on the part of the justice system to ensure that those who stand
accused bear the full weight of responsibility for the actions imputed to them.

In 1985, Richard Posner had this to say about the criminal justice system:

> The major function of criminal law in a capitalist society is to prevent
> people from bypassing the system of voluntary, compensated exchange –
> the 'market'. (Posner 1985, 1195)

In recent years, one could be forgiven for thinking that this had become
the ambition, not merely of the legal system, but of all the public services
as they are reconfigured to ready incapacitated citizens for involvement in
'voluntary compensated exchange'. In conjunction with this, the notion of
responsibility is used by some practitioners and commentators to restrict
the availability both of services and compassion, and to construct the client
as someone whose egregious behaviour emerges on purpose, thus meriting
punitive sanctions. Our observations here echo and extend those of Goode,
Greatbatch et al. (2004) and Lester and Tritter (2005).

We will illustrate these themes with material from practitioners and clients
in mental healthcare, as well as statements from policymakers and academics,
which tend toward the notion that in mental healthcare the citizen's actions
are under voluntary control and that they will respond to the prospect
of punishment. The emphasis on responsibility was seen by some of our
informants as a kind of justification for a reduced level of service and involved
the typification of some service users as 'timewasters'. Paradoxically, these
tendencies have occurred alongside the development of notions of 'service
user empowerment', yet clients (especially those with difficult or demanding
problems) are empowered merely to contend with more limited and more
punitive services.

The Origins of the Culpable Patient

The notion of individual responsibility is extremely elastic and it is this
versatility that contributes to its usefulness in discourses of mental healthcare,

as a means of undermining the status of both the client and the difficulties that they are experiencing. In the case of people who are 'sectioned' – that is, detained compulsorily under the Mental Health Act – the client by definition has had choice and responsibility removed from them. Yet, as Newnes and Radcliffe (2005) note and as we have observed ourselves, under the current regime they will be continually urged to 'take responsibility' and may well be prosecuted for behaviour that in a previous climate was not considered unusual when displayed by someone detained under the Mental Health Act. As Bjorklund (2004, 188) observes, the 'expectation that "the mentally ill" will attempt to control (i.e., take responsibility for) their behaviour despite the fact of their mental illness, is a pervasive feature of psychiatric approaches to the care and treatment of "the mentally ill".'

These debates are not new ones. Nineteenth-century psychiatrists such as James Cowles Pritchard and Henry Maudsley wrestled with concepts such as 'moral insanity' in which a person might do outrageous or bizarre things yet not appear to be insane in the more usual sense. The German psychiatrist J. L. Koch (1891) coined the term 'psychopathic' and was convinced that such 'inferiorities' were not true mental illness. These categories may be seen as precursors of some present day notions and today a curiously similar argument rages over the increasing number of people who are said to have 'borderline personality disorder' and who are believed to be capable of 'taking responsibility' if they wished (Brown and Crawford 2007). Our concern is that the ground is shifting and the net of 'individual responsibility' is being spread so as to enfold increasing numbers of people and deflect them away from services which might otherwise have benefited them but which are, as we have argued, increasingly difficult to access.

Changing Practice, Changing Culpabilities

The link between notions of responsibility and changes in the readiness with which service providers will administer services has been underscored by a number of conversations that we have had with practitioners over the previous five years or so. Mental health practitioners who qualified before the 1990s have spoken to us of the 'change in climate', of how a new generation of mental health professionals has been educated to accept ideas of individual responsibility uncritically, and of the brutality and inhumanity that they believe is arising from this. Some practitioners feel that, as a consequence, there has been an almost complete abdication of mental health professionals' responsibility to care for their clients. One general practitioner told us that he believed that 'old' psychiatry involved supporting people who couldn't take responsibility but mental health professionals are now washing their hands of such clients and another general practitioner observed that it is almost as if 'treatable mental illness' has been 'defined out of existence'.

The emphasis on personal responsibility harmonizes with a broader movement in government and public service that Wacquant (2007) characterized as 'neoliberal penality'. Ascribing a purported failure of self-control and responsibility on the part of marginalized people is, in this view, part and parcel of a move to treat them as culpable actors deserving of criminal sanction. If they know what they are doing with mischief in mind, then a punitive response rather than a therapeutic one is merited. As discourses of responsibility are implemented in therapeutic contexts, the vocabulary of motives attached to patients becomes conceived in forensic terms warranting a more punitive response. As Rose (2010, 84) notes, the trend of contemporary legal practice is toward 'the premise of the inescapability of moral responsibility and culpability'. Now, in combination with the tendency towards determinism in psychiatry which we have noted above, the moral responsibility of the culpable patient is not weakened, but rather is rendered more profound. The morally unacceptable conduct of the individual, says Rose, is more likely to be seen as indelibly inscribed, and not susceptible to rehabilitation, therapy or reform.

In addition to the slippage from framing clients and their troubles in terms of mental health to seeing their conduct in terms of personal – or even criminal – responsibility there is the vexed question of diagnosis itself. Diagnoses are often problematic, not least because the mental health service in one of the localities where we have undertaken research diagnoses a high proportion of clients with 'personality disorder'. Many of these clients subsequently received other diagnoses upon seeking help from services in other geographical areas. Their experiences as 'personality disordered' patients illustrate the imputation of moral responsibility particularly well in that it is accompanied by inferences that the person is wasting the time of practitioners, is being manipulative or is attention seeking (Brown and Crawford 2007).

The permeation of the notion into public policy that one can readily do something about one's status as an invalid, and the sense in which it is formulated as a matter of psychology, was illustrated by the comments of the then welfare minister Margaret Hodge, reported in the press in November 2005. Referring to proposals to use cognitive behaviour therapy to reduce the numbers of people claiming Incapacity Benefit for mental health problems, she maintained that if she encountered such difficulties she would consult a 'life coach', but the benefit claimants 'pull a sickie' (Hinsliff 2005). Leichter (2003) attributes the persistence of the idea of holding the individual responsible for their own health status to the emphasis in Western culture on individual rights and responsibilities and the diffusion of this into European cultures through the twentieth century. However, because of the financial problems and constraints faced by the NHS in the UK, economics nearly always enters the argument too – issues of whether the NHS can 'afford' to treat people who have been the architects of their own downfall are discussed (Walker 2006). Conversely, it is argued that 'taxpayers' (with the implication that in order to pay tax people must be employed) are seen as more worthy recipients of care and because they have putatively funded the NHS they are more fully entitled to care no matter how their ailments have been incurred (Edgar 2007).

Thinking about Responsibility in Mental Healthcare: Policies and Practitioners

The first hand material which appears in this chapter has been accumulated as a culmination of our three decades of involvement in mental healthcare as service users and carers, as well as our more recent academic interest in the field as researchers. The material that follows, with which we flesh out the theme of personal responsibility and how it has risen to prominence in mental healthcare, is therefore based on a number of different sources of information. It is informed by policy documents, such as the National Service Framework for Mental Health (Department of Health 1998, 1999), as well as its more recent updates (Appleby 2004, 2007). It is also informed by academic commentaries on policy changes in healthcare towards a foregrounding of service user perspectives (Appleby 2000; Carr 2007; Cowden and Singh 2007). Moreover, we have recently supplemented these sources with a series of interviews conducted with service users and a variety of practitioners including care assistants, nurses, occupational therapists, general practitioners and psychiatrists. These people were all connected with health and social care services, mostly in Wales. On reading the interview transcripts, policy documents and academic accounts, the notion of responsibility and its particular tensions in the field of mental healthcare emerged clearly.

The idea of moral judgments being made upon people with mental health problems is very well explored and documented (Leichter 2003; Olstead 2002). However, the manifestation in our own investigations was somewhat different. In line with Rose's (2010) observations, people in receipt of mental healthcare are not seen merely as 'bad' any more, but instead are seen as not exercising responsibility, whether their actions are distressing to others or to themselves. It is as if some service providers and policymakers believe that they could choose not to break the law, upset others, live in chaos, fail to support themselves and in some cases even to choose to stay alive, if only they would 'take responsibility'. In the field of mental health, such concepts are not confined to laypeople. One psychiatric social worker, the manager of a community mental health team, whilst discussing the difficulties of her job, told us that one of the biggest problems was that 'people think they have no responsibility...no responsibility to get better'.

This is aligned with trends observed elsewhere. Goode, Greatbatch et al. (2004) explored the idea of 'entitlement' to treatment among callers to NHS Direct, noting that individual responsibility for the health of 'empowered' patients acting as 'consumers' was promoted and was aligned with policy documents describing 'empowered' health consumers (Goode, Greatbatch et al. 2004, 211). There is much talk of 'empowering' 'service users' in mental health, but we suggest that the evidence indicates, as Freire (1973) stated, that the 'empowered' are not the same as the powerful. Twenty years ago in a British context, Cochrane (1989, 178) argued that 'in a situation of poverty, empowerment must of necessity take on a political meaning in the sense that the transformation of needs into rights is a sociopolitical process'. In the case of mental healthcare, his insights seem to have been extraordinarily prescient. He notes that 'In many ways the current pressure to "clientise" poor people is an effective form of control because they become categorised and therefore subdivided politically' (Cochrane 1989, 180). This, we contend, is what has happened to mental health 'service users'. They are 'clientized' rather than made powerful.

Campbell (1996, 224) observed that 'madpersons as empowered customers of services and madpersons as equal citizens are two quite different propositions'. Campbell (2001, 81) maintains that 'the great irony about mental health service user action in the past 15 years is that, while the position of service users within services has undoubtedly improved, the position of service users in society has deteriorated'. Whilst agreeing that 'empowered service users' are certainly not always treated as equal citizens outside of the mental health services, it is doubtful whether they are being appropriately respected within those services either. We have been told by one consultant psychiatrist that the model his own NHS Trust uses of service user involvement is 'purely tokenistic' and a consultant psychiatrist in another NHS Trust observed that 'there is a lot of tokenism about'.

The deaths of David Bennett, Roger Sylvester and Geoffrey Hodgkins among many others (Carvel 2006), as well as the numerous highly critical reports that have been compiled in recent years regarding the state of the UK mental health services (Wales Audit Office 2005; Healthcare Commission 2006), suggest that the clients of these services are not exerting much power at all. The New Labour government's Mental Health Act (2007) provided further evidence that people with mental health problems and their advocates have very little power. Paradoxically, the notion of the 'service user' has, through reinforcing notions of individualism and personal responsibility in mental health, restricted the material powers of these individuals. It 'clientizes' them or treats them as consumers, to the detriment of any more nuanced appreciation of the powers involved in keeping them away from the means of effecting change. In our experience, discourses emphasizing the view of services as something to be consumed are prevalent within the service users' movement itself. Notions of mental health as meaningful within a sociopolitical context or any radical analyzes of the power relations involved are relatively underdeveloped. This does not mean that users and the groups to which they affiliate are entirely without power, but rather it highlights how the problems, sites and forms of visibility are conceptualized and accorded significance. The key questions for us are how practitioners, policymakers and service users have posed and specified the problems of responsibility and the systems of action through which they have sought to enhance or impose it.

Consumption, Self-Determination and Victim Blaming

The individualization and responsibilization is detectable particularly through the focus in many conventional and complementary regimens upon consumption and personal healing. Olstead (2002, 636) analyzed media coverage of mental health self-help groups and found that the focus of the articles tended to be on individual healing, defining it as a personal problem, by the use of such phrases as 'encouraging one another' and 'self-determination', representing people as 'good' if they try and heal themselves. Olstead notes that the use of the phrase 'need to overcome' (2002, 636) reinforces the idea that mental illness is something over which people have control. As Olstead indicates, the language and concepts used in the media reports being scrutinized are indeed often the language and concepts used by many 'service user groups'. 'Empowerment' features frequently in the literature, yet the dominant discourses of service users themselves often revolve around individual 'healing', being 'strong' or being a 'survivor'. As Rose and Miller (2010) have remarked in a slightly different context, personal autonomy cast in these terms is not the opposite of state or political power, but a key term of its exercise. Our suspicion that there may be more to autonomy and empowerment than the straightforward exercise of personal powers was activated, for example, by hearing some mental health clients castigated by other mental health clients for 'not trying to get better'. One users' group that we know of vigorously promotes the use of 'complementary therapies'. Whilst clients may well gain a sense of personal benefit from treatments outside of the NHS or from treatments not considered 'mainstream', there may well be undertones of 'victim blaming' inherent in many such therapies, especially if they appear not to be having the desired effect (Coward 1989; Lowenberg 1989; Stacey 1997).

The past two decades have seen a growth in this is particular type of victim blaming. Indeed, commitments to individual empowerment are often closely aligned with complementary healing agendas (Hill 2003). Yet as well as blaming the victim, these tendencies are seen by some as representing a broader and more complex process of subjectification and personalization of public life (McClean 2005) and this itself is growing as a kind of rationality for rendering the personal and the social thinkable in such a way as to be amenable to medical and political deliberation (Rose and Miller 2010).

Goode, Greatbatch et al. (2004) explore the social relations that are being formed as professionals and 'users' adjust to the new health environment and note how as 'responsible' citizens whilst 'consuming' services, users are also judged as to whether they are being 'responsible' or 'irresponsible'. They observe that in healthcare discourse a species of 'timewaster' has emerged, the equivalent of the 'scrounger' in the welfare services. Timewaster files are being compiled on patients in some healthcare facilities (Gray 2006). This notion of clients as having the potential to waste the time of practitioners emerges in some unexpected places. For example, the idea of being a 'timewaster' emerged into the public domain in north Wales in a case when a mental health worker received a prison sentence for having a sexual relationship with an in-patient (BBC 2005). As part of the defence of his actions, the worker was reported as describing the patient to the police as a 'timewaster'. This might be unusual, but what is important here is how being a 'timewaster' contributes to a kind of political rationality. In other words, it is part of a morally coloured world view, grounded upon a particular kind of knowledge and made thinkable through language which can be deployed to devalue and dehumanize clients and deflect (in this case unsuccessfully) claims that they have been ill-treated.

An occupational therapist in an inpatient acute psychiatric unit that we interviewed spoke at length about the labeling of certain patients as 'timewasters'. He felt that it was an extension of another discourse formerly applied to some patients, namely that their symptoms were said to be 'behavioural'. He stated:

> What you found was that certain groups of patients were actually becoming an irritation and despised by health workers. If they were seen as...abdicating personal responsibility, then they would actually be seen as time wasters, taking up people's space, 'they're not really ill, I can't be bothered with people like this' and these were the sort of conversations that took place...when I started to get more senior in my own personal position...it became more and more apparent that people were actually failing to recognize a patient's actual illness...I noticed it was much more apparent with the group labeled 'personality disordered'.

This man believed that there has been an increased use of the term 'personality disorder' since he qualified twenty years ago:

> People who had previously been called bipolar, or schizophrenic or schizoaffective disorder would suddenly after years and years, it started to be said 'well I think there might be a touch of borderline' or whatever… I would say it started happening in the mid-90s…so the fact that somebody was a repeat, coming round and round and round, initially their chronicity was seen as the chronicity of illness, but eventually it was questioned as to whether it's the chronicity of illness or whether it was a personality trait that couldn't be made better. I think there was a genuine belief…but it was a belief that had been set up because of the paucity of treatment that had been given.

Goode, Greatbatch et al. (2004) describe how patients generally fear being labelled timewasters and use various criteria to demonstrate that they are 'deserving'. The impression painted by Goode, Greatbatch et al. is generally one of intimidated patients trying to justify their use of the healthcare system, although patients did become more assertive if they were accessing care for someone else. Lester and Tritter (2005) reported a variant on this among mental health clients when accessing services. Although the clients were already 'in the system', they maintained that accessing support, even in a crisis, was so difficult that various strategies were used, such as 'acting up' or enlisting other people whose opinion might carry weight, such as their vicar. We encountered similar tales of such strategies in our research. We also heard staff describing patients as 'manipulative' when patients were said to be 'pulling out all the stops' in a desperate attempt to access care. This reflects the struggle between funders, clinicians and patients that Goode, Greatbatch et al. (2004) also document, and indicates, as they suggest, that patients have not become empowered, they have just been given more responsibility.

One hospital had such a reputation for refusing to assist mental health clients, that a psychiatric social worker told us that even referrals from community practitioners had to be worded very carefully to ensure that psychiatrists could not easily refuse to treat the client. We were told that 'problems' arose with newly qualified community staff, or staff new to the region, who were not *au fait* with the wording needed on letters of referral to this hospital to elicit treatment for their clients.

Goode, Greatbatch et al. (2004) describe the terminology of healthcare professionals as they talk of 'appropriate' and 'inappropriate' use of services but fail to define what they mean. We have witnessed the confusion of clients when faced with such distinctions that they find difficult to map onto their own experience or their own sense of need. Goode, Greatbatch et al. (2004, 222–3) observe that consumers of health and welfare are now required not just to turn a critical gaze upon their bodies, 'but also on their own use of welfare services'. They also observe that the majority of their interviewees 'provided not so much a picture of empowered health consumers as that of…negotiating an identity of responsible health citizen' (Goode, Greatbatch et al. 2004, 228).

One of our informants, who had suffered from badly managed serious mental health problems with devastating consequences for many years, remembered very clearly being accused of not 'taking responsibility' for his own recovery. He compared his experience in climbing with that in mental healthcare:

> If I break my leg the A&E will reset it. Some comment may be made about how unsafe climbing is but they will still help me and treat me with care. I will be expected to exercise personal responsibility by following medical advice – leaving the plaster on for example. But I will not be expected to take personal responsibility for setting the leg that is broken. Is that dissimilar for expecting someone to take personal responsibility for fixing their life when significant parts of it have been so damaging?

We noticed an interesting phenomenon during our interviews with people involved with the mental health services – the idea of someone, who even by the standards of the service, was seriously distressed (sometimes sufficiently so as to have warranted involuntary hospitalization), still being deemed 'responsible'. We know of a case in which a patient detained under the Mental Health Act was prosecuted for calling the mental health unit manager a 'fat idiot'. This patient was deemed to be sufficiently irresponsible to be detained in hospital against her will and to be medicated against her will, yet was deemed fully responsible when she insulted a manager. We were told that, in this case, the police expressed the opinion that it would be ridiculous to charge the patient under such circumstances, but that the manager concerned and the clinical director of the mental health unit insisted that charges should be brought. Our investigations disclosed that the man who had been called a 'fat idiot' rang the police eight or nine times in the course of a single day to complain about the incident. Although the mental health unit involved became well known locally for such actions, their stance was far from unique and highlights the efforts made on the part of some organizations to deflect clients into the criminal justice system and away from mental health services. Whilst this might be considered unusual, it aligns with reports elsewhere of patients detained under the Mental Health Act encountering problems for not taking responsibility (Newnes and Radcliffe 2005).

Writing in the *Independent* in September 2005, Jeremy Walker, a psychiatric social worker, complained that the police are not more willing to arrest and charge patients when they are summoned to incidents at mental health facilities. In his view, arresting people has a remarkably prophylactic effect: 'If Christopher Clunis had been prosecuted for any of the serious offences he committed before killing Jonathan Zito, that tragic event might never have happened' (Walker 2005). Under this ideology, complete with its speculations and scare stories, to do other than prosecute clients who shout or have tantrums is, in Walker's terminology, 'patronizing' to them. In this way, relationships are established between the nature, character and causes of problems facing service providers. The distressed or angry client is not, in this view, living in tragic circumstances and committing trivial infringements, but is rather a potentially serious offender in the making. The infractions of the distressed and the uncertainty over their conduct are transformed into the 'risk' of more serious events in the future. There has been the highly publicized case of the young woman who, as was reported by the press, repeatedly attempted suicide and was given an ASBO preventing her from going near bodies of water, bridges, railway lines and multi-storey car parks (Morris 2005) and the case of the self-harmer who was imprisoned for threatening to injure herself in a department store (Herbert 2005). In the latter case, the judge was reported to have taken the unusual step of issuing a statement expressing his horror that he was being forced to send this woman to prison, as there was not a hospital bed available for her anywhere. In the case of the young woman who repeatedly attempted suicide, it seemed that it was the magistrates who were being punitive, as the health professionals involved did make their deep concern known.

Evidence is mounting that people with mental health problems are being prosecuted throughout England and Wales, attested to by the continuing high numbers of people with mental health problems in prison, despite the agreement of many experts and advisors that this is a bad idea. Charges are often pressed in the context of the 'zero tolerance' policy of threat to NHS staff (Condron 2007), but there is a very elastic definition of 'threat' being used. 'Threat' can mean sectioned patients shouting or swearing. Whether charges are pressed seems to be far more a function of the degree of rapport between the patient and the staff than any degree of risk. Two practitioners told us of working practices that regularly place vulnerable, inexperienced or insufficiently trained staff alone with potentially volatile clients, providing the very circumstances in which such incidents are likely. One psychiatric nurse stated explicitly 'this zero tolerance is making it worse'. The possibility of a physical altercation translates, through a logic of calculation, into a risk and thence into a threat susceptible to penal management and sanction.

Formulating Threat and Creating Culpability

In many of these cases where clients have been prosecuted, there seems to have been no discussion of the legal principle of *mens rea*, where the intentions and presumed responsibility of a person committing an offence can be called into question if they are mentally disordered. Even in cases where offenders were consigned to prison, this kind of challenge was often not mounted, nor does it even seem to have been mentioned in the court proceedings.

This is an example of how, even for mental health services, clients are seen as simultaneously rational and irrational in much the same way that they were reported to be in the Canadian media in Olstead's (2002) study. There has been much written about the way in which media representations influence beliefs about people with mental health problems in a way that is usually inconsistent with those clients' interests (Wahl 1995; Philo 1996). Olstead, after Foucault (1972, 1980), notes that the cultural significance of media representations activates certain forms of social power, but also influences the production of a discourse on mental illness 'that includes, but ultimately exceeds, media representations' (Olstead 2002, 641). The people employed to care for and support clients are indeed using these same discourses. We know of a case in which the manager of a mental health unit felt able to state, in the context of a patient's behaviour, that 'just because you're mad you don't have to be bad'. This manager presumably believed that behaviour he found objectionable was a matter of choice, rather than a symptom, paralleling Olstead's (2002) findings. In a suggestive conference paper, Thakkar and Kini (2009) noted that reporting events in hospital to the police was 'good for nursing morale' whether or not this resulted in a successful prosecution and that it was felt by staff that the arrival of the police to question an accused patient in itself was an effective deterrent.

This sense in which patients or clients are assumed to have a degree of voluntary control over their actions is also found in the other popular representations of the issue. For example, Olstead (2002) described the media as reporting that the mentally ill 'deliberately commit crimes' or were 'deliberately' entering prisons, the emphasis on 'deliberately', suggesting that they are fully responsible for their actions. Olstead notes that as far as these media reports are concerned, 'the juridical and medical criteria that mark the conceptual difference between who is considered mentally ill and who is criminal, falls away. What is achieved is the possibility of seeing mentally ill people as medically irrational, legally responsible and consequently, socially immoral' (2002, 634). On the basis of the interviews that we have carried out and on a number of legal cases, this appears also to be the situation presently facing many mental health service users in the UK. Time and again we have heard mental health professionals, particularly when discussing patients considered difficult, making comments such as 'they knew what they were doing when they did that'; 'they might be ill but they knew what they were doing' or 'that's personality not illness'. Staff felt able to make such comments without any formal discussion regarding the presumed intentions of the patient or *mens rea* having taken place. One mental health unit where prosecutions of patients were activated by staff for a variety of seemingly trivial reasons, seemed to have developed a culture among the staff where patients are nearly always viewed in this manner.

The area inside the patients head – the realm of intentions, desires and responsibility – is opened up as a site of governance. The threat of criminal sanction is therefore employed not to guarantee that untoward conduct will not result, but to set one of the terms under which the putatively calculating patient will exercise their will. One practitioner employed by this unit noted how the ground was shifting in terms of people being deemed responsible:

> If they genuinely think that someone is acting like that because of their illness then they would be very forgiving and very tolerant…they deserve treatment and they will be a nice person afterwards…[but] more and more people are being made responsible…even though they are deemed to be ill…it is the health service itself, the healthcare workers saying 'I want to press charges'…you get this trying to determine what is behaviour driven by their personality and what is driven by their mental illness.

The views of the staff also rub off onto those around them. The NHS Trust running this unit employed a community liaison police officer, who was, in conversation with us, very sensitive to the needs of psychiatric patients and clearly had a very good rapport with many of them. Yet on one occasion, this police officer told us that he'd just warned a sectioned patient who was constantly dialling 999 for bizarre reasons that if she continued to do this, she'd be prosecuted. We expressed surprise that he'd done this and he told us that the mental health staff had told him that the patients 'had to be made' to take responsibility. The notion of criminal sanction as potentially therapeutic in itself, whilst it may seem bizarre, has precedent in the literature. Not only in the comments of Walker (2005) above, but in earlier work by Miller and Maier (1987), the therapeutic role of prosecution was identified, especially if it was maintained that the behavior in question was impulsive and originated in 'character pathology'. Coyne (2002, 142) suggests that prosecution of patients is a 'defensible view'. Thus, there is a long-running strand of practitioner and academic opinion about the alleged benefits of prosecution to patient and practitioner.

The idea that people with mental health problems sufficiently serious to result in them being admitted to an acute ward should be exercising individual responsibility also often results in what Coyne (2002) calls 'managerial' sanctions, such as their being discharged and refused treatment for conditions that had obviously been deemed to warrant care and treatment only days earlier. One member of staff commented on this:

> They've been discharged for aggressive stances, aggressive behaviour, explosive behaviour, because of drinking, taking of illicit substances – to a certain extent you can understand it, but again you also get to recognize the difficulty of working in the mental health environment and trying to make people take responsibility for something that might actually be an addictive behaviour, or a reaction to voices…people are being sanctioned for behaviour that I would consider to be almost normal in the mental health setting…its incredibly unpleasant…but it is something that in mental health that I think you might have to be aware might happen.

This practitioner had a view regarding the type of client who was most likely to be told to take responsibility:

> The people who present as most difficult to the system, the service, are the ones who are most likely to be diagnosed as suffering personality disorder… they are the people who tend to be deemed as personality disordered who… have to take responsibility for themselves and their actions.

Perhaps it is unsurprising that in these financially austere times, the clients falling into such a category are the more demanding ones with multiple complaints – perhaps even 'dual diagnoses' – that do not fit neatly into a category that can be addressed with an 'evidence-based' intervention. Some commentators are increasingly concerned about this tendency. Davies (2004) has written about his suspicion that diagnoses such as personality disorder are being used as a flag of convenience to justify the refusal to treat such clients. Dalrymple (2005) has also documented the convenience of shifting diagnoses, stating that he has seen doctors perjure themselves in order to evade the responsibility of finding hospital beds for potential patients.

Dwyer (1998) notes that even where state funded provision is available, eligibility criteria are applied so as to yield a more stringent assessment of need. This was certainly reflected in the perceptions of some of our interviewees:

> INTERVIEWER: Do you think the discourse of individual responsibility is being used more often these days in mental health?

PRACTITIONER: Yes, and it is being used more punitively and judgmentally
and its being used as a screening process – it is actually being
given to junior doctors now on the basis of if this person
presents with this type of behaviour, don't admit them…

The difficulty in obtaining treatment from secondary services has led to an
expressed reluctance on the part of primary care staff to make referrals at
all. A general practitioner told us that he probably referred no more than
one person a year to the mental health services because he maintained that
referrals nearly always resulted in a letter to him stating that 'this patient
will not benefit from psychiatric input'. He discussed at length exactly how
psychiatrists now see their role: 'It's a long time since psychiatrists talked to
people', yet psychiatrists were also reluctant to take on their longstanding role
of addressing medication issues in mental health. Problems that were judged
to be treatable by medication were also, said our participant, being referred
back to general practitioners. Thus the purview of some mental health
professionals – the patients that they will consider accepting and treating –
appeared to be getting smaller and smaller. This is in stark contrast to the
heyday of radical critics of psychiatry. When Rosenhan and his colleagues
published their key paper 'On being sane in insane places' (Rosenhan 1973)
or when Thomas Szasz penned *The Myth of Mental Illness* (1974), the concern
was that an expanding therapeutic mission on the part of mental health
professionals was identifying more and more human experience as meriting
hospitalization, often on arbitrary grounds. Now however, the challenge facing
clients and potential clients is how to obtain a service in the first place, rather
than, for example, deflection or a visit from the police.

The Carer Who Needs to Take Responsibility

Carers in particular reveal worrying anecdotes concerning the level of need
that they felt obliged to demonstrate before being offered social support. In
north Wales, one woman appeared in the local paper when it transpired that,
after 20 years of caring full time for her now middle-aged son diagnosed with
schizophrenia, she had enrolled for a course at a local college. Her son was
forced to sleep in her car in the college car park while she was in lectures as
he could not be left alone at home (*Daily Post* 2004). The woman in question
disclosed to us that the 'useless' mental health services had refused to provide
any sort of support for her son despite his very severe and enduring problems.
He had been assessed as not being 'in need' of such support. In this case it was
the carer, the client's mother, who was continually told to 'take responsibility'
as she begged for help with her son.

We were told by a number of interviewees of suspicions that another way of denying people support and care was simply not to assess them at all. One of the authors witnessed an incident in which a woman requested an assessment for her ex-husband, a man with a diagnosis of schizophrenia, who was clearly having difficulties and had been making threats to his neighbours. The man's key worker told his former wife that the key worker had spent 'over an hour' with him that week, would not go out to see him again and that he would have to 'take responsibility' if he assaulted someone. The degree of harassment and aggression to which his ex-wife and the neighbours were subjected was ignored and we were interested to see that no support was forthcoming from the statutory services. Although, as this man's difficulties increased, a group of people from the local church did attempt to support him, unfortunately his problems continued; he was banned from the volunteer-run local mental health drop in centres because of his 'inappropriate' behaviour, as the voluntary sector also often requires individual 'responsibility' on the part of its clients. Vigilante action from the neighbours resulted in him leaving the village some months later, compounding his difficulties and transferring the problem elsewhere.

The emphasis on risk and risk assessment in professionals' engagement with clients is often a means of avoiding engagement, rather than identifying needs or actuarial hazards. In January 2011, a report by Healthcare Inspectorate Wales into the circumstances of the murder of 84-year-old Margaret Ford by her severely mentally ill son in 2009 noted that the process by which carers and family members had to contact the social and healthcare teams was 'frustrating and cumbersome', that access to emergency mental health assessment and care was 'inadequate and burdensome' and that 'insufficient regard' was given to an assessment of Mrs Ford's role as a carer for her son (BBC 2011c).

In comments sadly familiar to anyone who takes an interest in reports reviewing the care of mentally ill people after tragedies have occurred, Health Inspectorate Wales concluded that Mrs Ford's murder could not have been predicted, that there was 'little' to suggest that her son was a risk to others, that the mental health workers in the area faced 'significant' support and resource issues and that the care and treatment of Mrs Ford's son was 'not sufficiently robust'. On the day of the murder, a care team had visited Mrs Ford's house after her family had raised concerns about her son and Mrs Ford's daughter later made another call to a mental healthcare officer about his deteriorating condition (BBC 2011c). The case demonstrates the alignment of workers who were disinclined to see the potential for tragedy with the body allegedly in place to hold them to account. Their reluctance to act prompted the agreement of the regulatory body that the tragedy could not have been predicted, privileging

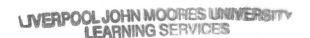

the inactivity of professionals over the freely expressed concerns of family members.

Situations involving desperate carers pleading for help were captured for us by the comments of a mental health practitioner:

> PRACTITIONER: If something does happen and it's can we get them into hospital? Why? Well they're starting to phone the neighbour, they're starting to irritate the doctor. Oh just tell them that they have to take responsibility, tell them that they can't phone at three in the morning...so these statements starts to be made, so that it's their fault, they've got to be responsible, they've got to stop doing these irritating things. If a wife or carer comes along and [details similar behaviour] it is seen as maybe you're being over fussy, maybe it's an over-engaged relationship – but when its demand on a service provider, it's seen as oh God they think they can just phone me up, who do they think they are.
>
> INTERVIEWER: The carers are expected to put up with a situation that the services can't?
>
> PRACTITIONER: I'd agree, that's something that I've seen over time. Again I think it's engendered by this belief that the person is responsible and should take responsibility and somehow cope themselves.

One of the mental health professionals that we interviewed summed up how views towards mental illness are changing:

> [Hospital employees] sort of expect people to be mentally ill...smelly and living in chaos...but it's OK to leave them like that because that's how they are...this is the discourse of personal responsibility...leaving people in illness seems to come from that belief – if you say they are responsible then that absolves you from your responsibility to help them.

We return now to the very articulate interviewee whom we quoted earlier in this chapter, who had experienced mental health problems for years and had regularly been told to 'take responsibility' by the mental health services. His perception was that this had caused him tremendous suffering – he had made a number of serious suicide attempts, his marriage broke up, he incurred a prison sentence and the successful business that he and his wife established lost a lot of money as a result of his frequent inability to run it effectively.

After finally receiving the help that he felt that he had needed for so long, he made some very insightful comments:

> I believe that the NHS has taken a stance throughout that period that they were blame free. I believe it is them, in fact, that has not taken responsibility and not provided adequate and appropriate help...the fact that I was sectioned at least three times and admitted to an acute unit probably another dozen times suggest that I was, at the very least, extremely distressed and in need of help... I have taken personal responsibility and worked hard to improve my situation because I have been given these two tools and support [a helpful consultant psychiatrist and therapist] with which to work... In conclusion I am like most other people and I try to do my best by myself. In their terms I take as much personal responsibility as I am able for my actions. When I have failed it is because I am not able and for the lack of a better description I am in a period of severe and acute distress or illness...to decline to help on the grounds of unwillingness to take personal responsibility...is a serious neglect of their duty. It is akin to leaving someone with a broken leg and saying that if he does not fix it himself he is not accepting personal responsibility and is therefore undeserving of help.

The effects of being expected to 'take responsibility' are not merely being felt by clients with mental health problems in relation to their healthcare. It is permeating many other areas of their lives as well. Early in the New Labour administration, Dwyer (1998, 494) observed that changes in welfare provision indicate a model in which state funded provision is 'dependent on an individual first agreeing to meet particular compulsory duties or patterns of behaviour'. From this, Dwyer argues that there is now a degree of conditionality involved in citizenship, welfare rights being conditional upon individuals accepting responsibility for their own destiny.

Conclusion

The events and tendencies that we have identified in this chapter do not necessarily all stem from a unified programme to make people responsible when they are in receipt of mental healthcare. As Rose and Miller (2010) remind us, welfare does contain a coherent mechanism which would enable the unfolding of a central plan, defined by powerful adherents of neoliberalism. The personnel, procedures, techniques and calculations that made up these activities are attached to specific locales and organizations: the hospitals, the community mental health teams, the courts and the justice system as a whole.

Nevertheless, by means of examples from our own work, reports of incidents from official bodies and the press and the resonance of this with a variety of research by other authors, we have attempted to sketch some of the processes through which the users of such services have come to be seen in terms of their ability or otherwise to take responsibility for themselves. The relatively large scale of mental health difficulties – broadly defined – means that the potential for usage of services is vast. Despite the increasingly robust claims that a third to one half of the population could suffer a mental health problem, this has been accompanied by a renewed focus on responsibility as a way of rendering the problems of disordered conduct and egregious demands on the part of the clientele of health services intelligible and manageable, and reduce the demand upon services. The responsible client, almost by definition, is less in need of care.

In the course of our involvement with mental health services as users, carers and researchers ourselves, we have had many conversations with practitioners and clients about 'individual responsibility', discussing the possible ideological or political reasons why, after generations of seeing the mentally ill as predominantly not responsible for their actions, we should now be encountering such a forceful promotion of the opposite notion – that they can and should 'take responsibility'.

This emphasis on responsibility has a good deal in common with the neoliberal drift in social policy and an increasingly penal approach to managing citizens who do not meet the criteria for full participation in the reconfigured post-industrial states of developed nations (Brown and Crawford 2007; Wacquant 2007, 2009). The 'penal societies' identified by Wacquant imprison people who are unable to cope with life under neoliberalism and do so by means of a transfer of institutional function from the welfare arm of the state to the penal one. The process of making those who do not cope with the changes in economic policy and social organization 'responsible' for their actions is an important part of formulating the issue so that punitive sanctions appear appropriate. In the UK, Wilson (2006) contends that prison serves to contain troublesome members of the population such as the mentally ill who now have little infrastructure to support them. Prison, in this view, has been reinvented and relegitimized as the functioning alternative to the former welfare state. Yet, as we have suggested, this punitive approach depends on a prior rearrangement in terms of how the service user's mind is conceptualized in terms of culpability and responsibility so that, rather than needing assistance, they are seen as somehow deliberately causing the problems within which they become entangled.

Neoliberalism in its broadest sense reactivates liberal principles, including a radical scepticism over the capacities of collective provision or political authorities to yield the best outcome, and vigilance over the attempts of policymakers and state agencies to govern, provide and act prudently in the public interest. The interface between service providers and service users in mental healthcare has been, as we have argued, sown with many examples of the practical implementation of this reconfiguration of government. The typification of sections of the population as disordered proceeds alongside a growing practical scepticism, in the face of an ever more austere unit of resource, of the deservingness of the service users themselves. Despite the way that their diseased identities are indelibly inscribed upon them as a result of putative disordered brains, dysregulated neurotransmitters or faulty genes, they are at the same time seen as active agents seeking to maximize their own advantage. They are believed to retain a capacity to calculate the relationship between actions and outcomes, so that in the face of expressed need they may be told to take responsibility for themselves and their loved ones and are, by virtue of being the legitimate locus of decisions about their own affairs, amenable to the threat of service withdrawal or criminal sanction, which as some authors document, may even make the care staff feel better.

This language of the entrepreneurial individual, who, despite his or her problems, is endowed with freedom and autonomy, has come to prevail in adjudications over questions of need, deservingness or service provision. It is this which continues to inflate prisons with people showing signs of mental distress and confusion, because some people will inevitably not be able to 'take responsibility' as mandated by the state, no matter how severe the sanctions.

Chapter Six

RESPONSIBILITY IN THERAPY
AND THE THERAPEUTIC STATE

Introduction: Individualizing Responsibilities

In the previous chapter we described how, under the guise of getting clients to 'take responsibility', the statutory mental health services had redefined their purview so as to limit the eligibility for help of a great many potential clients and their problems. Despite this retraction of care and the urging of the individual to take responsibility, it is however possible to see expansions of the medical or therapeutic world view into many other areas. We have already discussed this expansion in the form of screening and vigilance over health concerns in the physical realm in earlier chapters. The state and a variety of medical and public health agencies have taken on an expanding role as arbiters of risk where health is concerned. Governmental agencies and professional bodies alike counsel against the dangers of sex, knives with points, alcohol consumption and salt intake. Yet as we have shown earlier, there is a systematic devolution of risk and risk responsibility towards the individual. As the process of responsibilization proceeds it is the individual rather than the collective who bears the weight of these hazards and who is enjoined to 'take responsibility' for doing something about it.

In coming to an understanding of the therapeutic state and the implications that this has for responsibility, the legal scholar Helen Reece (2000, 70) reminds us how the idea of responsibility has itself been transformed – 'responsible behaviour has shifted to a way of being, a mode of thought'. The 'individual is judged, not by what he does but by how profoundly he has thought about what he does' and 'shows his responsibility by the attitude with which he approaches the decision'. Throughout the contemporary sociopolitical landscape there is a tendency to valorize thoughtful responsibility. It may not necessarily result in individuals making the kinds of decisions that follow yesterday's understandings of right and wrong, but it involves making them with due self-awareness.

Responsibility Humanized: Psychotherapy and the Responsible Individual

This combination of self-awareness and responsibility was most conspicuous in the past in mid-twentieth-century incarnations of psychotherapy and counselling. There is more than a casual affinity between the responsibility urged upon citizens in the contemporary era and that which was urged upon the therapy-seeking middle classes in the United States in the middle years of the twentieth century.

The strong tendency in psychotherapy to urge responsibility upon the client was central to the project of counselling itself, according to one influential figure in the development of UK counselling, Richard Nelson-Jones:

> The ultimate goal of counseling is to help clients towards taking effective responsibility for their own self-realizing. (Nelson-Jones 1979, 152)

Allied to this notion is that in being more responsible, one becomes more fully oneself, as if responsibility were the natural state of human beings:

> Therapists argue that the purpose of psychotherapy is to help the patient become more autonomous in their choices – that their choices represent their 'real' selves. This may mean that the person has to take responsibility for feelings and thoughts that they find uncomfortable, and which they may not have anticipated when they started the psychotherapy process. (Adshead 2008, 225)

For James Overholser, one of the risks in clients becoming aware of theories of mental distress which emphasize possible biological or cultural factors is that these 'may reduce the client's feelings of personal responsibility for change'. Instead, 'it is more helpful to cultivate attributions for personal responsibility for change, growth, and maturation' (Overholser 2005, 369).

This then is the stuff of responsibility notions in the literature on psychotherapy in the present. However, the genealogy of the idea goes back rather further than this. This strong emphasis on responsibility in counselling and psychotherapy owes a great deal to Fritz Perls, (1893–1970) in whose work assuming responsibility for the self is elevated to a high priority, over and above that of, for example, responsibilities for others. In approaches influenced by this kind of thinking, responsibility is seen as an important precursor to any kind of progress. In *Existential Psychotherapy*, Irvin Yalom (1980, 286), says 'In order to change one must first assume responsibility'. The theme of getting workshop participants to 'take responsibility' was also central to the so-called 'est' (Erhard Seminars Training) movement of the 1970s. Yet, as many commentators such as Yalom (1980) noted, the way in which participants and volunteer helpers were encouraged to give up their autonomy and subject themselves to a meticulous discipline seemed to be the very antithesis of assuming responsibility. Responsibility has to be exercised in the right way according to the edicts of the movement's leaders or it did not qualify as responsibility at all. Yet at the same time, across all these fields of endeavour, the therapist or group facilitator is at pains to stress that he or she has no responsibility for the clients or participants. In this view, shedding responsibility for anybody else is vital for the therapist and Perls advised that:

> The therapist has three immediate tasks: to recognize how the patient tries to get support from others rather than provide his own, to avoid getting sucked in and taking care of the patient and to know what to do with the patient's manipulative behaviour. (Perls, Hefferline et al. 1951, 139)

The project of responsibilization in therapy was not borne primarily from compassion. Rather, it stems from an impulse to force the client to assimilate or 'take responsibility for' all the undesirable things that might be going on in his or her social world. Whilst asserting that he had broken in significant respects from psychoanalysis, Perls was preoccupied with the psychoanalytic notion of 'projection'. Virtually everything his clients or workshop participants saw in the human world around them was to him a projection of some undesired part of the self, originating from an unwillingness to 'take responsibility'.

> We are not willing to take the responsibility that we are critical, so we project criticism onto others. We don't want to take responsibility for being discriminating, so we project it outside and then we live in fear of being rejected. And one of the most important responsibilities is to take responsibility for our projections and become what we project. (Perls, Hefferline et al. 1951, 217)

In this way, the individual and his or her 'projections' are at the centre of the topography and whatever they may understand about the social world is merely a projection of their own deficiencies and limitations. Whilst in the original formulation of Perls the therapist is absolved of responsibility, this nevertheless lays out more or less endless opportunities for intervention. The self, with appropriate professional help, can be reconstructed as one which is marked by responsibilities and it is the therapist's or facilitator's role to extend this into the variegated areas of a person's life. Even more significantly, once the process of responsibilization has been activated, the process may more or less be self-propelled: 'group members will recognize their own responsibility for learning and for moving themselves and each other toward optimal mental and relational health' (Bender and Ewashen 2000, 307).

Despite the break that the humanistic movement claimed to have made from psychoanalysis, psychodynamic thinkers were adroit at harnessing the discourse of responsibility to characterize the way in which the newly responsibilized client would be liberated from inner restrictions. Schafer (1976) described the neurotic restrictedness in which one feels oneself to be determined by ego-dystonic drives, thoughts and feelings as the result of a defensive self-alienation. In this process, one's motives and actions are not recognized as one's own and hence no responsibility for them is taken in an effort to avoid conflicts. Hence, psychoanalysis aims for patients to own these alienated parts of their lives once more and take responsibility for them.

Thus, via the inner topographies of self which have been laid out, the opportunity has been afforded for the construction of a self through the techniques associated with a liberal mentality of rule that valorizes self-reliance and responsibility in an uncertain world. As we have seen earlier, the political state that Rose (1999) calls 'advanced liberalism' promotes the need to adopt an entrepreneurial approach to one's identity, to manage one's own risks (O'Malley 2004), to be innovative, adaptive and most importantly, responsible. The so-called 'humanistic' psychologies which informed therapy, counselling, personal growth and the quest toward 'self-actualization' are aligned with this later movement, away from collective approaches to social problems and towards a reconfigured entrepreneurial self, capable of transcending welfare. In both humanistic psychology and under advanced liberalism, the new responsible, resilient self is a state that has to be achieved with professional intervention and advice, and one which is involved in constant struggle or processing, rather than taken as natural or allowed to develop on its own.

This is not to imply that policymakers have deliberately plundered the esoteria of the therapeutic and humanistic psychologies for ideas. Far from it: the ideas embedded in the current preoccupation with 'nudging' people towards more politically desirable behaviour, the development of happiness agendas, wellbeing measures and the recasting of citizenship in terms of responsibilities are regularly described as if they were new discoveries on the part of ministers and opinion leaders. Rather, what we are discussing is a mindset that makes possible particular ways of thinking about people and thinking about ourselves. This then becomes sedimented into a variety of other media such as self-help literature, public policy and practical common sense on a piecemeal basis and without any formal plan.

Nevertheless, the processes that we are discussing share important confluences with thinking in public health, social policy and risk management. The ideas in psychotherapy and counselling have much in common with what Greco (1993) calls a 'duty to be well'. The contemporary urge towards responsibility is part of a move to 'empowerment' that aims to propel citizens away from 'dependence' on professionals towards resilience and self-reliance.

This trend has become very obvious in the wake of the UK coalition government's determination to reduce public spending. The duties expected of citizens include not only duties to themselves but duties to others. The case of young carers provides an illustration of this trend. Coalition children's minister Tim Loughton was reported in the press in October 2011 as expressing concern about whether current welfare policies would adequately support young people caring for a family member. Said Loughton, if 'young carers were no longer able to provide care this could result in considerably greater costs being passed on to the NHS or children's social care' (Ramesh 2011, 6). The discovery and valorization of cadres of responsible young carers is also proceeding apace in our own area of residence, north Wales. The newsletter of Gwynedd County Council, *Newyddion*, has a history of stressing the services that the council provides, yet the autumn 2010 edition took a new direction. A front page feature entitled 'An inspiration to us all' described how a local 13-year-old girl makes 'an amazing contribution' to our society 'by giving much of her time to helping her parents to care for her older sister… who has severe learning disabilities'. The story details how the teenager has to rise early to ensure that the house is safe to prevent her sister from harming herself; how she washes, feeds, dresses her sister and keeps her occupied; how she doesn't have time to do her own homework or go to after-school activities and how some children at her school 'don't understand'. The story mentions that there are four siblings in this family. The teenager in this story is obviously admirable but one can only wonder why this family is not receiving more assistance from Gwynedd Council, rather than the council simply hailing their daughter as an inspiration to us all.

The same issue of *Newyddion* also reported on a local consultation on health and care services, with examples of (anonymous) comments allegedly made by service users at the consultation. Comments included 'services should not make you dependent – we can help ourselves and we should be helped to do this'. The winter 2010 edition of *Newyddion* ran a feature reporting comments made by local people who had attended an Older Peoples Conference, one of the featured comments being 'I believe that as a society we depend too much on public services like the Council or government. I would like to see the community itself looking out for each other, especially as people get older.'

What is striking here is that, although there are indeed many fiercely independent people living in this region no matter what their material condition, politically Gwynedd Council is dominated by Plaid Cymru and this type of relentlessly individualistic 'fend for yourselves' discourse had not previously been used. Residents of Gwynedd previously in receipt of social care services were certainly not overindulged; in 2008 Gwynedd Social Services had been the subject of a highly critical review (Wales Audit Office 2008) and there was much concern that, far from 'depending too much' on public services, many people were not receiving the basic level of support to which legislation entitled them.

This is but one example, yet it is emblematic of a wider trend in policy, politics and service provision. The harder problems of how to provide services and enhance living standards as well as adjudicate between competing interests and demands, are abandoned and instead the public are encouraged towards greater self-reliance and to enhance their ability to cope with uncertainty. This theme of coping with change and uncertainty and substituting self-reliance for use of (usually public) services has been adumbrated in a variety of self-help volumes and aspects of popular culture too.

Thriving on Uncertainty: Privileging Feelings in an Era of Austerity

The responsible, innovative and enterprising citizen is thus also more able to withstand the shocks and grasp the opportunities presented in the risk society. To aid the individual, as well as a range of therapies through which responsibility is enjoined, the last couple of decades have seen a plethora of new managerial and life skills texts for adapting the self to uncertainty. These include Peters' *Thriving on Chaos* (1987) and Covey's *The Seven Habits of Highly Effective People* (1989). These have now been joined by fashionable self-instruction manuals elaborating the techniques of resilience: *The Power of Resilience: Achieving Balance, Confidence, and Personal Strength in Your Life* (Brooks and Goldstein 2006), *The Resilience Factor: 7 Keys to Finding Your Inner Strength and Overcoming Life's Hurdles* (Reivich and Shatte 2002) and *The Resiliency Advantage: Master Change, Thrive Under Pressure and Bounce Back From Setbacks* (Siebert 2005). As with the psychotherapeutic maxims that we have described above, the material hardships visited upon the individual are not seen in themselves to be significant, nor do they even necessarily have an independent existence. What is important in this view is how the individual responds to them.

This might at first seem to be at odds with the overall project of neoliberalism dominated by concerns with the international movement of capital, ensuring the flexibility of labour markets and creating opportunities for investors.

This retreat into the subjective qualities of the social environment might seem to represent a flight away from the economic considerations that are said to govern policy.

To make sense of this apparent disjuncture, to enable us to see the links between these apparently contradictory processes and examine how they are linked, let us turn to a distinction made by Pierre Bourdieu (1999) in *Acts of Resistance*. Here, Bourdieu distinguishes between what he calls the 'right hand' and the 'left hand' of the state. The right hand of the state refers to those aspects of government concerned with military, policing and security issues, with prisons and with the distribution of wealth in favour of elite groups. Counterposed to this is 'the left hand of the state… the so-called spending ministries which are the trace, within the state, of the social struggles of the past' (Bourdieu 1999, 2). Typically it is the left hand of the state that is concerned with the matters of health, education and wellbeing that have come about through struggles on the part of the labour movement, those concerned with women's rights and the institutionalization of philanthropy. If the left hand of the state is concerned with the therapeutic and subjective aspects of the state, it may do this relatively independently of the economically hard-nosed right hand. For as Bourdieu sees it, the 'right hand…no longer knows…what the left hand does…[and] does not want to pay for it' (1999, 2).

Yet over the last few years there has been a rapprochement between the two hands of the state. The right hand and left hand seem to have been working in symbiosis, as if their interests were not in conflict. Those aspects of government which might once have been concerned with the wellbeing of the citizenry through investment in education and social welfare have developed an interest in phenomena such as wellbeing and happiness as subjective phenomena as well as – or instead of – the amelioration of material hardship.

Under the new coalition government, ministers have been heard to say that the economy measured in terms of the extent of fiscal activity – gross domestic product (GDP), international flows of capital – is relatively unimportant. What is more vital, it is suggested, is subjective wellbeing. This variant of wellbeing is conceived of as being relatively independent of income or wealth. Minister for universities and science David Willetts stated:

> What really matters is whether you feel that you belong, whether you are able to pursue personal goals in your life, and the strength of your relationships with others. Family, neighbourhood and nationhood all matter to us. (Willetts 2010, 38)

Wellbeing, says Willetts, has to do with the pursuit of external goals and happiness comes as a by-product of this. The imagery is determinedly nostalgic, replete with ideas about materially austere but interpersonally warm communities, full of people doing things for one another, with the sense that it all serves some higher purpose. In one sense, the left hand of the state is shrinking as there are recorded declines in children's centres, after school clubs, Connexions offices for young people, youth programmes, home visits for elderly people and so on. What has happened is that the left hand activities have been refocused into a therapeutic state and, moreover, one that is much more attuned to the needs of the right hand.

Therapeutic States: The Left Hand in the Service of the Right

The current preoccupation of David Cameron, David Willetts and many others in government with issues of happiness and wellbeing represent the latest flourishing of what has been termed the 'therapeutic state'. It is to this idea that we now turn to explore further how individualism and responsibility have become so deeply inscribed in the body politic. The phrase 'therapeutic state' has a long currency and has served as the title for books by Thomas Szasz (1984) and James Nolan (1998). It is to the latter that we now turn to examine how therapeutic concepts and ambitions have come to be built into the heart of social and political life. By way of this digression we will return to the contemporary interest in wellbeing and happiness in UK politics and show how the left hand functions of the state are becoming more closely aligned with right hand agendas.

Although published over a decade ago, Nolan's *Therapeutic State* makes a number of observations which are curiously prescient of the twenty-first century. For example, Nolan (1998, 2) describes how in America

> the therapeutic perspective has become a taken-for-granted part of everyday life. It provides culture with a set of symbols and codes that determine the boundaries of moral life.

In the therapeutic state, the individual is placed at the centre of the moral order. In place of older forms of moral authority, such as a higher spiritual power or a covenantal community to adjudicate on moral matters, the therapeutic ethos establishes the self as the touchstone of personal and moral life. Whereas earlier accounts of socialization and education had stressed the value of adapting the growing individual to the family and broader social order, with the development of self-psychology through the twentieth century it was increasingly felt that any constraints imposed by social obligations and conventions were oppressive and damaging. Instead, personal liberation, emancipation and self-actualization were formulated as key values.

The therapeutic ethos that Nolan sees as permeating cultural, public and occupational life is conspicuously self-referencing, rather than for example, referencing any broader collective entities such as the family or community.

In tandem with this focus on the self, Nolan maintains that there has developed what he calls, following Alasdair MacIntyre (1981), an 'emotivist ethic', such that an emphasis on emotions has come to play a central role in which truth is seen as bound up with sentiment or feeling, rather than through reasoning. The citizen as an active political agent thus recedes from view and is replaced by one who emotes and expresses freely, for to do so otherwise is to be in denial or dishonest. Emotions serve as the means by which one should make decisions, for relating to others and for understanding oneself. This does not mean that everyone in developed nations feels and acts this way all the time. Rather, argues Nolan, this is becoming the most readily available means in which our moral referencing and self-understanding can be conceived. Emotions denote authenticity, as when the former UK prime minister Gordon Brown cried in a television interview discussing the death of his daughter or when Bill Clinton as US president was overcome with waves of emotion.

For the general mass of citizenry, rather than emerging from the individual *ab initio*, these trajectories towards self-fulfillment and emotional expressiveness require a particular kind of pastoral attention. Thus, Nolan points to the significance of the new 'priestly class' of psychologists, psychiatrists and mental health professionals. They constitute impressive numbers in the American labour force and have assumed a degree of authority in helping individuals make sense of themselves and the social world. As well as professional assistance, a variety of voluntary and lay groups often conceived along the lines of the successful Alcoholics Anonymous model, cater to those who have defined themselves as suffering from disorders as diverse as compulsive shopping, being a 'workaholic' (a term which itself is freighted with implicit theories as to the underlying mechanisms), a sex addict, a debtor, a gambler or an overeater. Even if no problem can be identified with the individual themselves, a romantic partner or family member who is afflicted can mean that the individual is 'codependent' and thus merits inclusion as a sufferer from some sort of 'disease'. These disorders bring with them a whole apparatus of fellowship meetings, courses, committees, self-help reading matter and organized systems of social relations such as buddying, befriending and sponsoring, forming a curious new variant of what used to be called 'civil society'.

The American Psychiatric Association, which periodically publishes the *Diagnostic and Statistical Manual of Mental Disorders*, is understandably more circumspect about this proliferation of disorders. Despite vigorous lobbying, it has not included codependency among the disorders it defines and specifies.

Yet. at the same time, it is a key document in making everyday experiences and human variations into 'disorders'. Shyness or a desire for solitude might be 'avoidant personality disorder', an overinflated sense of one's own worth or conceit might represent 'narcissistic personality disorder' and anxiety and misery at the loss of a job might represent 'adjustment disorder with anxious mood'. Both medically sanctioned and voluntarily assumed illness identities are a type of social currency in this view, via a process akin to what Jean Bethke Elshtain (1995) calls a 'politics of displacement', such that concepts like sickness, disease, addiction and recovery come to be universally intelligible cultural and moral reference points.

Yet, despite this self-scrutiny, this emotivism and this meticulous cataloguing of the disorders of the individual, it is surprising how robust political and economic systems appear to be. Nolan points to the way that a therapeutic culture – indeed, a therapeutic state – may actually be providing capitalism with what it needs to preserve itself:

> The therapeutic orientation provides a personalized remedy to a highly impersonal, rationalized, bureaucratic system, but without fundamentally altering the system. (Nolan 1998, 20)

It is this that secures the relationship between the left hand and right hand of the state. The economic and disciplinary matters of statecraft remain intact and largely unscrutinized, whilst the emotionality itself is deployed, described, managed and subject to therapeutic interventions. These therapeutic left hand activities are in the process of jockeying for position with old-fashioned social welfare directed towards ameliorating poverty, improving education or preventing disease. It seems as if the material conditions are less important than how the citizens might feel about themselves.

The ascendancy of the emotivist self offers new entrepreneurial opportunities and the individual who is particularly adroit within the emotional economy is hailed by such new opportunities. The emotions one undergoes offer a way of credentialling the self. Emotivism provides a supplement to more traditional moral codes and symbols. Nolan sees this as being akin to a sort of Bourdieusian 'cultural capital'. Offering oneself as an emoting, distressed or damaged individual has a kind of exchange value. This may be in terms of the credence given to one's claims as someone who is suffering or who is struggling with adversity, or even in terms of the additional help or benefits which may be available. Nolan (1998, 19) speaks of the 'stronger currency found in therapeutic ideals', which enables people to bolster their claims.

Narratives of distress or damage have become commonplace among 'graduation success stories' of some universities. The reporting of such stories on university websites or the local media manifestly pays tribute to students who have overcome considerable obstacles and succeeded. Yet in more recent years 'graduation stories despite disadvantage' have become extraordinarily personal, mentioning students' experiences of sexual abuse, severe mental illness, homelessness or institutional care. The description of such graduates as suffering or damaged people is usually more extensive than the text concerning their academic success. It is paradoxical that the graduation story is ostensibly a tale of how the graduate has put their distressing past behind them and is moving into a bright new future, yet what is preserved for posterity is the trauma and unhappiness that they experienced until recently; it is after all their suffering that made them newsworthy.

Suffering as capital can be seen in the way in which people tell the stories of their lives, or of one another's. The idea of the 'misery memoir' came to the fore in the 1990s, yet it represents a modern flourishing of a much earlier form of storytelling. Some commentators see the forerunner of contemporary misery memoirs in the reminiscences of Siegfried Sassoon in his *Memoirs of a Fox-Hunting Man* (1928) or *Memoirs of an Infantry Officer* (1930). There are many examples in the contemporary era. Among the best known is Frank McCourt's *Angela's Ashes* (1996) in which he describes growing up in poverty in Ireland in the 1930s and 1940s, detailing hunger, the death of siblings and the tribulations attached to having an alcoholic father. David Pelzer's *A Child Called It* (1995) describes his abuse at the hands of his alcoholic mother and his father's apathy. These stories and many others like them have, through the 1990s and early twenty-first century, been part and parcel of the publishing industry.

So great is the impulse to develop the claims to personal frailty, misery, squalor and deprivation, that the claims made in supposedly autobiographical books are sometimes difficult to sustain in the light of more thorough investigation. James Frey in *A Million Little Pieces* (2003) describes alcoholism, crack addiction and the suicide of his girlfriend. Yet the veracity of his claims was challenged from a number of quarters, not least Oprah Winfrey, whose book club had originally endorsed the title, and *Freakonomics* author Steven Levitt. A similar story attaches to a book entitled *Love and Consequences: A Memoir of Hope and Survival* (Jones 2008) in which the protagonist claimed to have had a childhood in foster care and to have been an active member of a gang from an early age, carrying firearms and dealing in drugs. Subsequent disclosures by the author's sister revealed that instead she had grown up in an affluent suburb with her biological parents, never having been fostered or been a drug dealer. Such was the embarrassment suffered by the publisher Riverhead Books, that all copies remaining unsold were withdrawn.

These few examples should suffice to illustrate the capital that can be drawn out of misery, deprivation and even law breaking on the part of the protagonist or author – so much so that some authors have sought to embellish otherwise unremarkable childhoods and early adult lives in order to address the vogue for misery memoirs. Published book length works, especially those netting substantial royalties for their authors, represent only a tiny fraction of the overall stock of human misery. Nevertheless, they illustrate Nolan's point that there is a kind of capital to be accumulated from the unhappiness one can claim to have suffered.

This process is evident in a more demotic form in popular magazines such as the UK's *Take a Break*. On its website it proclaims that 'We're interested in your lives. Love and betrayal, loss and sin'. The process is made easier with the provision of a web form to outline the story and the submitter's contact details, so that 'one of our trained writers will get back to you'. If selected for publication the fee 'can easily reach four figures'.[1] Thus, those who may not have the inclination to acquire a contract for a book length manuscript from a publisher can still enjoy the opportunity to turn misery into capital. As Furedi (2002, 221) argues:

> The state of vulnerability has acquired formidable social prestige. The victim is no longer someone to be pitied – it is a status to which many aspire. As an object of cultural empathy, the victim serves as an affirmation that human existence represents a state of vulnerability.

Since the publication of Nolan's book, the development of the therapeutic state has continued. Recently, the UK coalition government proposed a 'happiness index', announced by prime minister David Cameron. Cameron was reported to say:

> If I thought this was woolly and insubstantial, I wouldn't be bothering with it. To those who say this sounds like a distraction from the serious business of government, I say finding out what will improve lives and acting on it is the serious business of government. (Grice 2010, 24)

Rather than voicing something distinctive to the coalition government, Cameron was continuing a direction in policy that had been set in train sometime earlier. Adviser to the previous New Labour government, Richard Layard (2007), promoted the view that it should be the purpose of schools to promote the learning of happiness skills and to develop good and happy

---

1 http://www.takeabreak.co.uk/send-us-your-story (accessed 25 December 2010).

people. To this end he endorses a programme known as the Penn Resiliency Project. This was devised by

> Martin Seligman, the founder of 'positive psychology'. In it, fifteen 11-year-old students spend 18 classroom hours on such issues as understanding their own emotions and those of others, and developing concern for others. They are taught by one teacher, who has been trained in the method through eight hours of online self-study and 10 days of face-to-face training. (Layard 2007, 20)

The meticulous quantification of the size of the groups, the hours of training for the instructors and the classroom hours involved for the students seems curiously at odds with the more nebulous curriculum content involved. What would happen if it was an hour more or less? The enthusiasm is for measurable encroachments into the curriculum and the impetus to introduce measurable improvements in children's wellbeing – reducing their rates of depression by 'one half'. Layard is similarly laudatory about the notion of 'values schools' where children are taught to control their emotions by means of familiarizing them with 'uplifting ideas' and silent reflection (Farrer 2000). Similarly, it is important from his point of view that teachers have 'clear values' and that it is valuable to 'train up the emotions that support moral action' (Layard 2007, 21). He endorses the idea pioneered in California, of 'compassion gyms' where the mind can be trained in compassion in the same way as the body can be trained and its fitness enhanced. As we can see here, a curiously physical metaphor for moral and political processes is extended. Compassion can be exercised – literally. The qualities needed to succeed in the therapeutic state and live out the ethic of emotivism can and should be trained from an early age. Such is the intensity of physical metaphor here that one can say that Layard truly has a vision of the body politic.

Measuring Wellbeing: Happiness and Trust on a Shoestring

At the coalition government's request, the Office for National Statistics has begun developing a policy with regard to measuring wellbeing in future investigations of the issues. Here too it is possible to detect a drift of argument away from material factors in wellbeing and towards psychosocial aspects:

> Subjective wellbeing data have previously demonstrated that unemployment is associated with significantly lower levels of life satisfaction and this effect is largely because of the lack of social engagement rather than the loss of income. Therefore, these data can

and have been used by policy makers to develop 'active welfare policies
that prioritise fast-tracking the unemployed back to employment
rather than just boosting their financial support'. (Office for National
Statistics 2010, 34, citing Donovan and Halpern 2002)

In line with the therapeutic state thesis, the Office for National Statistics
document performs a manoeuvre that we have outlined above, that of
reducing the significance or value of those aspects of the left hand of the state
that involve spending, and enhancing those aspects that involve a focus on
interior variables such as wellbeing:

> The main advantage of asking people to assess their own wellbeing is
> that paternalism (prescriptive questions that assume certain things are
> good or bad for wellbeing) can be avoided and people's thoughts and
> feelings are placed at the centre of policy. (Office for National Statistics
> 2010, 34)

The Office for National Statistics, in the same report, points to the fact that
questions about aspects of wellbeing have been asked regularly in a number
of sample surveys that it administers and endorses the idea of teaching
wellbeing in schools (Bacon, Brophy et al. 2010). The wellbeing agenda has
transcended the older ideas about democracy in which people might respond
to the vision or policies of candidates or parties and vote accordingly. Now
it is the government's job to massage or even to manipulate the electorate's
wellbeing.

   The Institute for Government's (2010) 'Mindspace' paper set about
outlining strategies to achieve this. A great deal of emphasis in the document
concerns the 'framing' of initiatives so as to yield greater public acceptability.
For example, one should avoid talking about 'behaviour change' (2010, 63),
as this will make the proposed manipulation less attractive. Maybe, say the
authors, the government should take the lead even with unpopular policies,
citing the London congestion charge, which became more accepted after it
was introduced than before.

   As commentators such as Brendan O'Neill (2010) have remarked, this
approach to the process of government represents a downscaling of politics.
Once politics may have been concerned with how we might achieve prosperity,
how we might adjudicate between competing interest groups or institutions, or
even ambitiously unfold visions of what a 'good society' might look like. Now
it has been scaled back considerably so as to focus on behaviour and interior
constructs such as wellbeing, whose subjective nature and whose relative
independence from 'right hand' economic variables is seen as a positive

advantage. The territories of government are shifting away from the hard problems of economics – which are increasingly difficult for governments to solve anyway – towards new theatres of operation. The 'body politic' is inverted so that the sphere of action is inside the individual citizen's subjective territory.

This has gone hand in hand with a more general psychologization of politics. From the cliff-face rise in terms such as self-esteem, trauma, stress and counselling in public discourse (Furedi 2003), to the cultivation of a 'vulnerable subject' in political language (McLaughlin 2010), a great many commentators have pointed to the growing pervasiveness of a personalized, interior language in public debate and policy circles. As part of this psychologization, alongside the question of 'responsibility', the issue of trust has been extensively debated. This is not a coincidence. In order to comply with the 'Mindspace' oriented attempts at manipulation, the populace must subscribe to the notion that institutions and policymakers are trustworthy. Indeed, commentators on the contemporary political scene such as Anthony Seldon (2010) are apt to conceptualize the citizen as a trust seeking resource object. It is no surprise in relation to this that there is a new found reliance on the explanatory powers of psychological processes in contemporary politics. Commentators are increasingly likely to talk of the malaise in contemporary politics and policy in terms of interior psychological qualities. For example:

> Politics as we know it has ended because people no longer trust or respect politicians. (Morrison 2010, 22)

Or, as veteran journalist Polly Toynbee put it, quoting the British Social Attitudes survey:

> British Social Attitudes shows trust in politicians at an all-time low. First MPs' expenses, and now the torn up manifestos have left 40% saying they 'almost never' trust governments to put the public interest first. (Toynbee 2010, 31)

Layard (2007, 19) places trust at the centre of politics and policy too, pointing to a UNICEF survey that

> asked 11–15-year-olds 'Are most of your classmates kind and helpful?' 70% or more said 'yes' in Scandinavian countries, but the figures were considerably lower for some other countries: 53% in the United States, 46% in Russia and 43% in Britain.

The loss of trust is seen as regrettable, as if matters would be better if only ordinary people were to trust both one another as well as politicians and experts. The trust proposed is often a one way process. The apparent distrust expressed by a variety of policies directed towards the populace, including surveillance, inspection, regulation and control is less emphasized compared to the apparently lamentable lack of trust displayed by the populace themselves.

Ordinary people's trust is seen as something that is in crisis. The idea that trust is a value that is desirable in civic life and is something which can be cultivated by judicious social policies is the subject of a volume by Anthony Seldon (2010). Seldon, who became famous as the biographer of former UK prime minister Tony Blair, is also master of the prestigious independent school Wellington College and was famously involved in not only making it coeducational but also introducing happiness classes based on positive psychology.

Somewhat paradoxically, Seldon sees the solution to declining levels of trust as involving greater regulation and state intervention in the lives of citizens. Journalists, in his view, cannot be trusted to self-regulate, so he argues for enhanced powers for the Press Complaints Commission and for reporters to take journalism exams. He proposes that some people should be dissuaded from having children until they are 'ready'. Schools should play a much greater part in the upbringing of children and young adults should face a compulsory period of service in order to become more trustworthy citizens. This might involve activities such as looking after the elderly, picking up litter and repairing fences, as well as 'emotional intelligence' classes. The duty to be trusting and the responsibility for being trustworthy Seldon says are incumbent upon all.

The sense that something could and should be done about trust as a political priority is part and parcel of the psychologization of politics and a further manifestation of the tendencies that we identified in earlier chapters for policy and politics to be directed towards the governance of conduct. The project of governance in Seldon and Layard's ambitions goes even further, so as to address not only conduct, but the configuration of consciousness itself. Whilst the ethic of emotivism has enabled emotionality to feature ever more strongly in the public domain, what is emerging is not so much a raw emotionality, but rather a cultivated and expert mediated version of the sentiments. It is as if people cannot be trusted to have feelings all of their own, but rather require training in order to deploy emotions properly in their personal and social lives and cultivate an appropriately trusting attitude toward politicians and a variety of forms of expertise.

This management of the emotions which is identified as being so desirable is often subsumed under headings such as 'emotional literacy' or 'emotional intelligence', and has gained purchase with *bien pensants* such as Layard and Seldon as well as the political class. For some time now, the idea of emotional intelligence has figured prominently in the literature of self-fulfilment and self-realization. In the words of one of its proponents, Daniel Goleman, it 'refers to the capacity for recognising our own feelings and those of others, for motivating ourselves, and for managing emotions well in ourselves and in our relationships' (Goleman 1998, 317).

This construct is interesting because of the readiness with which it has been grasped over the last couple of decades and the extent to which it is urged upon both public and private organizations and on ordinary citizens as a facilitator of 'success'. Yet the enthusiasm for this construct also extends the reach of an ambition towards the interior management of the citizen and a desire to ensure that the emotional life of the employees of a firm, the pupils of a school or the population as a whole has a degree of consistency and pre-approved predictability.

The desirability of an alignment between the individual citizen's emotional life and that of a broader consensus is made explicit in the case of commonly used measures of so-called emotional intelligence. For example, the Mayer–Salovey–Caruso Emotional Intelligence Test asks respondents questions such as 'What moods might be helpful to feel when meeting in-laws for the first time?', asks them to predict the response of an employee faced with increasing work demands and asks them to identify emotions represented in a face. Respondents can be scored in relation either to group norms derived from administering the questionnaire to a large pool of respondents or their scores can be compared to those of 'emotion experts'. Whilst the authors of these kinds of measures are apt to see them as measuring something akin to intelligence, maybe they are merely measuring conformity (Roberts, Zeidner et al. 2001) or the ability to align one's judgments with that of others or cultural commonplaces such as one might encounter in a soap opera, situation comedy or feel-good movie.

But there is something else awry in the emotional intelligence project. The measurement of emotional intelligence by means of predicting in hypothetical scenarios and rating photographs in this way suggests a value attached to leaping to judgment. One must do so to answer the questions at all. Yet, in the complex world of human affairs, judgments needed are infinitely more subtle and may usefully be more circumspect. A smiling face may indicate happiness, yet a moment's reflection may suggest examples of people whose public persona was markedly at odds with the misery they inflicted on their families, whose smile might accompany an intent to deceive or even clinical depression. It is true that a man might be overwhelmed by increasing work demands, but this involves subscribing to a notion of human nature which sees personal capacities as finite and apt to be depleted. Absent from this logic is any sense that people can triumph over challenges through assiduous work or ingenuity. The templates of emotional life for which the 'emotionally intelligent' person instinctively reaches are relentlessly trite, hastily assumed and imbued with a pessimistic view of human nature that emphasizes vulnerability at the expense of fortitude or stoicism.

Medicalizing Ourselves, Mitigating Responsibility

The independence, self-reliance and trust that citizens are enjoined to experience has limits. There are contradictions between the self-reliance and entrepreneurialism demanded on the one hand, with the cultivation of vulnerability that is predisposed on the other. In any event, the individual is posited as being the site of a kind of dialectic between responsibility on one side and vulnerability on the other. The demands for independence are counterposed by demands that the individual seek professional assistance and advice where matters of health, wellbeing and happiness are concerned. The vulnerability that citizens are enjoined to experience may be at odds with the overarching sense of responsibility.

The problem faced by individuals labouring under such conditions is how the imputation of responsibility for oneself, one's family life, employability and parenting proficiency can be mitigated in the event of its not meeting the standards demanded. If the emotivism transcends the boundaries of what is 'healthy' and becomes excessive, or the self is destabilized to the extent that the desiderata of good citizenship cannot merely be recovered by taking responsibility, one is confronted with an explanatory problem. More immediately, one is confronted with the problem of how one's livelihood and one's identity project as a whole may be sustained.

One pathway through this apparent impasse is provided by the notion of illness. If a problem is defined as medical rather than personal or psychosocial it relieves the individual of responsibility for overcoming it, but also confers new responsibilities for seeking help from appropriately qualified people. The term 'medicalization' was coined to describe the expanding mission of the health professions to define an increasing number of everyday conditions and experiences as medical matters. Originally, in the 1960s and 1970s, social critics such as Ivan Illich, Michel Foucault, R. D. Laing, Thomas Szasz and others raised concerns about medical concepts, procedures and power tending to supplant alternative ways of characterizing and explaining human problems. Yet this kind of medicalization is only part of the story in the present era. Rather than healthcare professionals continually expanding their ambit, the impetus is often from patients or would-be patients themselves, keen to acquire a medical warrant for their problems.

The growing tendency to interpret failures of the project of the self under neoliberalism in medical terms has been noted by a number of students of medicalization. Conrad in *The Medicalization of Society* (Conrad 2007, 3) notes that:

'Medicalization' describes a process by which nonmedical problems become defined and treated as medical problems, usually in terms of illness and disorders.

Moreover:

The key to medicalization is definition. That is, a problem is defined in medical terms, described using medical language, understood through the adoption of a medical framework, or 'treated' with medical intervention. (Conrad 2007, 5)

Conrad describes the task of medicalization as proceeding via four processes, namely extension, expansion, enhancement and continuity. The process of *extension* is illustrated by Conrad in terms of the ways in which men's bodies and problems have increasingly come to be seen as meriting medical surveillance and control. Women's bodies, especially their reproductive health, have for a long while been addressed by both healthcare practitioners and women themselves in this way. Recently, however, the medicalization project has been extended to men's bodies, by means of attention to 'conditions' such as the 'andropause', baldness and erectile dysfunction. The *expansion* of medical categories over time is demonstrated, says Conrad, by the incorporation of adults into the diagnostic system of attention deficit hyperactivity disorder (ADHD). The process of *enhancement* is exemplified by the way in which drugs that are approved to treat one condition may come to be used as enhancements for others. Whereas the examples illustrating extension, expansion and enhancement show the growth of medicalization, the fourth process, *continuity*, is illuminated with an example which, at first glance, might serve to illustrate an opposite process of demedicalization. Since its removal from the American Psychiatric Association's *Diagnostic and Statistical Manual* in 1973, homosexuality might appear to represent one of only a few examples of demedicalization. However, Conrad argues that several recent shifts are facilitating a process of remedicalizing homosexuality. Conrad avers, for example, that the emergence of a 'born gay' philosophy in many US gay communities shows the growing popularity of a biological model of homosexuality.

In the event of people falling into a contested or morally problematic category, a medical definition of the situation can confer some advantages.

In Schubert, Hansen et al.'s (2009) study of drug-dependent adults with a diagnosis of ADHD, the category 'ADHD patient' was used by interviewees to claim membership of a 'morally neutral' category as opposed to 'illicit amphetamine user'. This manoeuvre relieves the patient from responsibility (Schubert, Hansen et al. 2009, 499).

This example from Schubert et al. is but one item in a raft of processes which seek to identify failures in the entrepreneurial project of the self as medical problems. As Holmqvist (2009) argues, social issues are likely nowadays to be understood and managed through medical models and processes. Mathieu's (1993) study of the medical anthropology of homelessness in New York revealed that:

> Politicians and the press consistently linked homelessness with mental illness, thus medicalizing a socioeconomic problem. Although some homeless people were also mentally ill, most people were not and had become homeless because of decreased low-income housing, declining real wages, unemployment, and cuts in government benefits. (Mathieu 1993, 170)

Mathieu's study suggests how attention may be refocused from social issues towards personal problems. The medicalization of homelessness in New York served to delegitimize any account of the plight of homeless people that saw them as victims of political and economic shifts during the Reagan administration. Thus, the ground was cleared for the unfolding of an explanation in terms of individual pathology and deficiency, diverting attention from possible suggestions that structural causes of growing poverty in the US might be culpable.

In a related study, Holmqvist (2009) shows how people out of work in Sweden are apt to be classified as suffering from some sort of illness or disability as a way of facilitating their access to different kinds of support and also, crucially, as a way of explaining their unemployed status. 'The phenomenon of formally classifying unemployed people as "disabled" illustrates how a modern welfare state tries to "solve" social issues by treating them as personal problems' (Holmqvist 2009, 417). Identifying the source of the problem as a disability makes 'the unemployed individual responsible for his or her situation by claiming that he or she is sick or disabled and therefore needs to be rehabilitated, reformed and activated' (Holmqvist 2009, 408).

Within the discussion of medicalization, the idea that pharmaceutical companies attempt to create and shape markets for their products has been well rehearsed (Angell 2004; Petersen 2008). The expansion of the pharmaceutical industry especially since 1980 and its influence over the academic literature of medicine and debates concerning health in the public sphere are well known. A different perspective on this process is given by Tone (2009), who points instead to the way in which there was an audience for pharmaceutical advertising because the public was receptive. Consumer demand, Tone maintains, led pharmaceutical firms toward more aggressive marketing and to attempts to manipulate prescribing physicians. Especially where tranquilizers were concerned, the practice in the US ensured that the majority of prescriptions were issued by ordinary family physicians rather than specialist psychiatrists. The prescription of minor tranquilizers and many common antidepressants is something that can be done by non-specialist doctors, often in response to patient demand, a practice that started with the tranquilizing drug Miltown in the 1950s and continued with direct-to-consumer advertising in the present era. The majority of psychotropic medication is in the hands of patients and general practitioners rather than mental health specialists and is available to ameliorate the everyday experiences of distress.

Conclusions

The notion of responsibility is one which has a substantial and persuasive pedigree in psychotherapy, counselling and self-help movements that served to offer it as a means to liberation and place it on the public agenda. Under the development of the therapeutic state, the responsibility placed on the individual has expanded. It is now enjoined upon citizens at a level that seems to parody the style of group facilitators in Werner Erhardt's est groups. The ability to take responsibility has been posed in therapy and in politics as a kind of liberation, an opportunity to reclaim alienated parts of one's life and enjoy a sense of integrated wholeness. As Rose and Miller (2010) have pointed out, there is a curious alignment between this rise of the individualizing and responsibilizing tendency in the psychology of self-actualization and personal growth in the postwar period and the transformations in politics in the present. The very interpermeability between notions in psychology and ideas in the political sphere has facilitated the translation of notions in therapy to ideas in policy and politics. Where they are exhibited, the responsibilities exercised by citizens – as carers, as people seeking to live independently of public services, as individuals who can resiliently cope with uncertainty and 'thrive on chaos' – are celebrated. Policymakers are apt to see the quality of the national experience – happiness, wellbeing and responsible participation in 'big societies' as key to the wellbeing of the nation state itself and the therapeutic perspective has become firmly embedded in the art of statecraft. The presence of emotion in public figures, the detection and sustenance of disorders in everyday life and the ready availability of concepts such as sickness, addiction and recovery as intelligible cultural and moral reference points are elements in what has been called 'emotivism' in public life, and this in part helps to deflect attention away from the possibility of more material or thoroughgoing political attempts to enhance life quality. There is even a bizarre sense in which suffering, distress or hard luck stories are themselves a kind of social capital and can yield lucrative book contracts and a kind of celebrity in its own right. The presence of material on happiness, emotional life and wellbeing in the educational curriculum is endorsed by public figures such as Anthony Seldon and Lord Layard, and the Office for National Statistics' efforts to measure wellbeing requires that 'thoughts and feelings are placed at the centre of policy'. The hard problems of economics, managing prosperity or adjudicating between competing interests or institutions are put on one side in favour of an ever more meticulous engagement with the putative inner world of the citizen. Solutions to social problems are thus personalized and individualized rather than collectivized in the therapeutic state. Moreover, this approach is focused, not on the creation of bonds between citizens on the basis of shared experiences of adversity, but instead emphasizes professionalized relationships based on expertise and an unequal relationship between expert and citizen. This may take the form of tutelary relationships in formal therapy or through coaching, or may be manifested as attempts at a policy level to treat problems as psychological issues through the deployment of initiatives to increase trust, responsibility and emotional intelligence at a societal level. The spread of these kinds of initiatives has proceeded at the same time as a gradual stripping away of the traditional Keynesian 'left hand' initiatives relating to education, health and welfare. Thus whilst responsibility, trust and 'emotional intelligence' are encouraged for the responsible citizen, there is comparatively less attention given in many of these policy discourses to the social structural aspects of the problem.

One form of escape available to the individual from the relentless thrust of responsibility is towards a medical definition of the problem suffered. Medicalization under the therapeutic state offers a means of redefining the situation, so that one's malaise may be understood as placing one beyond the reach of certain kinds of responsibility and one's problems outside one's own volition. Rather than the mission creep of health professionals and drug companies, medicalization is sometimes urged upon the health professions by clients and consumers themselves, activated and trained through the variegated self-help and therapy movements and schooled in the disciplines of the therapeutic state. Problems of a variety of kinds – unemployment, homelessness, a disengagement from politics or a perceived lack of trust – are likely to be seen in terms that are personalized, individualized and interpreted through the lens of psychology or medicine.

From the 1940s to the present, responsibility has been reformulated as a matter over which the 'psy' disciplines have dominion. Rather than a construct within jurisprudence, responsibility is to do with a capacity to think, reflect, overcome and capitalize upon trauma and an ability to see oneself in the vocabularies of interiority, emotion and personal growth. The path here is not entirely straightforward and involves the citizen negotiating a number of tensions and dilemmas. On the one hand, the responsible citizen is self-reliant, but on the other responsibility is something that the individual can take only after having been subject to the expert intervention of therapists, self-help specialists or classroom wellbeing interventions. On the one hand, the process of personal growth towards responsibility requires a relentless vigilance, but at the same time being able to show one's suffering or achieve a medical-sounding warrant for one's condition or situation yields a social cachet too. Responsibility is not an end point or something that can be achieved once and for all, but needs to be continually struggled for, carefully husbanded and scrupulously exercised. Responsibility is a lifetime's work.

Chapter Seven

THE PUNITIVE TURN IN PUBLIC SERVICES: COERCING RESPONSIBILITY

Introduction: Responsibilization and Coercion

So far, we have been considering the way in which new developments in the organization of civil society and the delivery of public services have fostered new kinds of consciousness and new conceptions of the citizen. In this chapter, we will consider some aspects of what Garland (2001) has termed the 'new punitiveness' and examine the implications of this for the development of responsibility and responsibilization. The implication that the individual, if not deemed responsible, trustworthy or reassuring, will be subject to punitive sanction underlies a great many policies, items of legislation and a range of civil orders such as Anti-Social Behaviour Orders (ASBOs) which may be applied to the recalcitrant citizen. In addition, with a vigorous programme of new legislation, the previous New Labour government introduced a variety of novel ways in which civil and criminal sanction could be applied to the populace. Moreover, as we shall explore through the issue of housing, a range of new actors have been enlisted in the quest to encourage and enforce responsibility in different civil spheres. Once again, the process is coercive as well as facilitative, because failures to meet the requirements placed upon the individual may result in eviction or ineligibility for a new tenancy. The culture of audit, inspection and sanction has been applied not only to individual clients or service users, but to practitioners and professionals in a variety of public service roles. This does not necessarily guarantee a better service for the client, but brings ever greater numbers of professionals into the web of scrutiny.

New Punitiveness: Extending the Reach of Carceral Systems

The rise in prison populations in many developed nations, especially the US and the UK, has been remarked upon by many commentators (Garland 2001; Wacquant 2009), and the argument has been made with some persuasiveness that the process and practice of incarceration is central to statecraft in late modernity. Whilst this critical scrutiny of penal policy has been mostly directed at the US, many commentators also highlight the example of the UK as one of the foremost European nations embracing punitive measures (Gottschalk 2009) such that penal policy is subtly remaking the notion of citizenship itself.

Since a historic low point in the early 1970s, by the early years of the twenty-first century the US prisoner population increased by more than six-fold (Manza and Uggen 2006, 95). By this time, the US had incarcerated a higher proportion of its people than any other country. By 2005, seven million people – or one in every 32 adults – were either incarcerated or under some other form of state supervision, such as parole or probation (Glaze and Bonczar 2006).

In the UK too, crime control policy was framed as a zero-sum game between victims and offenders (Newburn 2007, 459) in which benefits to victims correspond to pain for offenders. In the 2005 election campaign, the Conservative opposition signalled its willingness to raise the incarceration rates of England and Wales to 200 per 100,000 – or about double the average for Western Europe. That this proposal 'passed without comment' is a 'sign of how far such rhetorical pledges have become normalized' in England and Wales (Downes 2007, 103).

Some of the debates about penal policy can be seen unfolding locally in specific parts of the UK. For the last few years, there has been a campaign to support the building of a prison in north Wales. Much of the campaign has been conducted in public meetings and in the media. Although it is admitted that north Wales is not a region that experiences high levels of serious crime, the campaigners maintain that there is an absolute necessity for a prison in north Wales, because people in the region currently have to serve their sentences in south Wales or England. This involves transferring them to prisons many miles away and their families having to travel great distances to visit them. It is also argued that there is no facility for Welsh-speaking prisoners. This is all true, but what interested us is that the campaigners initially made much of the alleged economic benefits and employment that a prison would bring to the area. Elsewhere, especially based on experience in the US, doubts were being expressed about the viability of prison building programmes to revitalize the economies of rural areas (Mosher, Hooks et al. 2007; Gilmore 2007). In north Wales, a number of local residents and business people who opposed the building of a prison began a vigorous counter-campaign and conjured up images of horrified tourists arriving to enjoy the scenery and visit Caernarfon castle, only to encounter a prison as they entered the town. The debate intensified and on 24 November 2010 the *Daily Post* ran an article entitled 'N Wales jail is a "human right"', in which local MP Elfyn Llwyd argued that it is a matter of 'human rights' that prisoners from north Wales are located near their communities and families. The notion of human rights is used in a particularly flexible manner here, and was adduced seamlessly to the case for incarceration. By focusing on criminal justice solutions to questions of human rights and economic development, this apparently progressive move aligns itself with a raft of tough sanctions, many of which are at odds with the interests of the region.

Ap Gruffudd (2007) found that Welsh-speaking prisoners incarcerated in English prisons were routinely denied their legal right to speak Welsh to each other or to conduct telephone calls in Welsh on the grounds that this constituted a security risk – monolingual English-speaking prison officers expressed fears that prisoners could be planning their escape in Welsh. We should explain to readers unfamiliar with Wales that there are a small number of prisoners whose English is not good and who communicate far more easily in Welsh and it is likely that they want to discuss rather more mundane concerns in Welsh than escaping. Yet instead of any attempt to use existing legislation to secure language rights for Welsh-speaking prisoners, the difficulties that they experience are deployed as part of the justification for an addition to the penal state itself and the carceral economy is positioned as a major contributor to economic life in the region. It was proposed at one point that the prison in north Wales should be a 'titan prison', with a capacity for 2,500 prisoners. It is difficult to believe that there are 2,500 Welsh speakers in need of incarceration or indeed that imprisoning 2,500 residents of Wales would be an advance of anybody's human rights. The key feature here is that incarceration itself is so readily recruited to the policy themes of human rights and economic and social regeneration. The carceral state 'shapes individual civic capacities, efficacy, and perceptions of government' (Weaver and Lerman 2010, 829).

This carceral enthusiasm on the part of politicians in the UK and reformers seeking to revitalize regional economies has recently been punctuated by the publication by the coalition government of a green paper entitled 'Breaking the Cycle' (Ministry of Justice 2010), that proposes a greater use of noncustodial approaches and rehabilitation in an effort to reduce the population in prison. Its launch was accompanied by speeches and published interviews with its main sponsor, Kenneth Clarke: 'It's loopy to think that locking everyone up will solve crime' (Sylvester and Thompson 2010, 42). Yet the carceral impulse is nevertheless strong in government and in press opinion. The *Daily Telegraph* bemoaned the fact that under existing policy

more than 56,000 of the most hardened offenders were not put behind bars last year. They included 4,000 violent criminals, 94 sex offenders and almost 3,000 burglars. Even though the courts are less willing to jail serial offenders, their numbers are on the rise. (Whitehead 2010a, 10)

Any proposals to reduce prison numbers or reduce tariff sentences for those pleading guilty at the outset was said to represent a 'betrayal' of those bereaved as a result of violent crime (Barrett and Hennessy 2010, 4). As Simon (2007, 110) states, an important strand in public debate has 'defined the crime victim as an idealized political subject…whose circumstances and experiences have come to stand for the general good'. Thus, despite the green paper proposals, the emphasis upon punitive sanction is still strong, is in harmony with rising prison numbers and represents a dominant frame through which contemporary crises of authority are understood.

Many critics point to the deepening disparity between rich and poor, and it is in this contexts that policymakers and 'professional managers of unease' (Bigo 2002) have attempted to enhance the insecurities of the public (Garland 2001), as well as build electoral support through calls for harsher sentences (Reiman 2004) with a view to enhancing their popularity in impending elections (Pratt 2005a; Simon, 2007). This movement forms part of a so-called 'new punitiveness' characterized by an increasing 'tolerance for brutalizing penal sanctions and prison conditions that some 30 years ago or so would surely have been quite unthinkable' (Pratt 2005b, xi). These developments have proceeded in parallel with increased social marginalization, rising rates of poverty (Beckett and Western 2001; Wacquant 2009) and broad cultural shifts towards increasing social divisions and more exclusionary forms of society (Young 1999).

Thus, through the 1990s and early twenty-first century, we have been faced with the spectacle of political parties vying with each other to propose ever larger increases in the number of people who can be incarcerated. But the headline figures alone represent only a small part of the way in which public life has been recast in terms of enforcement and punishment. It means that, for significant swathes of the population, the justice system (including the police) comes to be their major means of interacting with the state (Weaver and Lerman 2010). It means that in the process of government, the 'technologies, discourses, and metaphors of crime and criminal justice' (Simon 2007, 4) have been migrating to other institutions and public policies that are not immediately connected with fighting crime.

Behind the process of imprisonment on both sides of the Atlantic lie what Fine and Ruglis (2009, 20) call 'circuits and consequences of dispossession', such that people who are imprisoned are usually there as part of a longstanding trajectory through a variety of health, welfare and educational deprivations, and dispossessions. Poor young people especially tend to migrate out of the educational system and into 'carceral corners of the public sphere'. Even for those who are not inside them, prisons cast a long shadow over the topography of inequality. This is what Carlen and Tombs (2006, 338) mean when they use the term 'cultural economy of imprisonment', which they explain refers to

> the iconic status historically given to the prison's mythic powers to protect governments and citizens against threats to the body politic as a result of law breaking, unemployment, immigration, visible marks of exclusion from citizenship and threatening otherness of any other kind.

Similarly, in his key text *Discipline and Punish*, Foucault (1977) uses the concept of the carceral to describe the distribution and normalization of disciplinary techniques throughout the landscape of social institutions. He saw this as culminating in the emergence of a 'panoptic society of which incarceration is the omnipresent armature' (Foucault 1977, 301). However, writing in the middle years of the twentieth century and not living to see the large scale incarceration of the present day, Foucault 'failed to realize that, far from being fated to recede into the societal background to make room for dispersed disciplines, the prison was here to stay right alongside them – indeed, it was about to grow to proportions never before envisioned' (Wacquant 2002, 384).

As the prison population grew, Piche and Larsen (2010) remind us that governments began a dismantling of the welfare state, driven by a rationale which stressed fiscal conservatism, individualism and market fundamentalism (Giroux 2009). This resulted in a retraction of services, including mental health facilities and in the US at least, and a reduction in funding for community based alternatives to incarceration. This left many people who might previously have benefited from services fending for themselves (Scull 1984). Under these circumstances, community based interventions often acted as a larger pipeline to conduct the mentally ill and poor to prison (Collins 2008).

At the same time as the punitive ethos has been extended and enhanced, there has been a growing call for a more assertive response to 'the scourge of antisocial behaviour and its corrosive effect on our society' so as to 'beat the scum ruling our streets' (Jones 2010, 13). This was accompanied by documents such as 'Antisocial behaviour: Stop the rot' from Her Majesty's Inspector of Constabulary (2010a), which advocated assertive early interventions by the police in relation to reports of anti-social behaviour:

> Managing ASB is crucial to sustaining the vitality and confidence of communities. Untreated ASB acts like a magnet for other crime and disorder problems and areas can quite easily tip into a spiral of economic and social decline. (HMIC 2010a, 12)

In this sense, HMIC is orienting to anti-social behaviour via the lens of 'broken windows' theory, originated by Wilson and Kelling (1982) and popularized by the former New York City police chief William Bratton. The idea is that small indices of neighbourhood disorder such as incivility, graffiti and the eponymous broken windows themselves, if checked early enough, can lead to reductions in crime as a whole. This approach has been discredited on intellectual and empirical grounds (Wacquant 2009), but has a life beyond its formal underpinnings, as well as a seductive commonsensical quality. Moreover, it helps extend the rationale for more assertive policing of neighbourhoods where disorder may occur. This is entirely in line with the broken windows approach – in Wilson and Kelling's original account the main target of intervention was not windows at all, but people: 'disreputable or obstreperous or unpredictable people: panhandlers, drunks, addicts, rowdy teenagers, prostitutes, loiterers, the mentally disturbed' (Wilson and Kelling 1982, 29).

Punitiveness beyond the Prison: Extending the Reach of Sanctions

In recent years in the UK there has been a new focus on maintaining order by means of penalties which operate outside the court service. As well as the police, a variety of officials are empowered to levy on the spot fines and fixed penalty notices. Such non-court options were deployed in around 567,000 or 'nearly half' of the 1.3 million recorded offences in 2009–10 (Whitehead 2010b), a development favourably regarded by HMIC (2010b) with a view to streamlining the justice system so that increasing numbers of citizens can more efficiently be brought within its penal compass.

This expansion of the penal remit sits alongside the growth in other more subtle forms of governance. As we have seen, the processes of governmentality are concerned with the creation of a contemporary sense of self (Caplan and Torpey 2001). From the point of view of Foucault and others such as Rose (1999) and Dean (1999), who developed Foucault's ideas, the process of producing subjects' identities, subjectivities and sense of self is a vital part of enabling governance to be accomplished at a distance. This kind of governance at a distance or regulation of conduct is seen as a central mechanism of rule under advanced liberalism (Foucault 1991; Lemke 2001). As the technologies of the self are deployed, power need not be manifested directly to enforce compliance onto the subjects. Instead, the mechanism of rule is manifested through technologies of the self, in that subjects are implicated and enrolled in forms of self-government, aligning the self-regulating capacities of subjects to dominant norms (Dean 1999). In this view, the people over whom power is exercised are not passive recipients of the dictates of the powerful, but are active agents in reconstructing and shaping their identities themselves. Yet under advanced liberalism, this self-government and investment in the self goes alongside, and is undergirded by, a more penal and coercive process. This involves sanctions for a variety of forms of conduct which may be deemed anti-social or undesirable.

There are, of course, preferred norms of citizenship promulgated through speeches, policy documents and via the agencies of the state, but what is crucial is how people position themselves in relation to these. For example, Clark (2006, 211) reports that his young son asked him 'is there a law saying you have to eat five fruit and vegetables every day?' In examples like this it is possible to see the blurring between advice, exhortation and legal obligation which yields a self-imposed sense of obligation, irrespective of the likelihood of formal sanction.

A result of both the legislation created and the means by which it is enforced has been to create a citizen who is perpetually at risk of penalty. A variety of activities which might never have been considered as matters for penalty before have been brought under the remit of officials empowered to impose them. A glance through the previous year's newspapers provides a variety of examples. Whilst these do not present a picture of the operation of justice in the round, and focus on examples which might appear absurd, unfair or which have been successfully challenged, it is instructive to see the kinds of conduct which are tackled at the leading edge of this legislative advance. Amongst other things, press reports in the UK describe new on the spot fines of £110 to penalize those who do not sort their rubbish for recycling appropriately (Derbyshire 2010) – this is £30 more than the typical penalty for shoplifting. The former lord mayor of Leicester was reported to be fined £80 by one of the litter wardens he had been instrumental in employing for dropping a cigarette (*Daily Telegraph* 2010a). A retired solicitor was arrested and issued with a fixed penalty notice for attempting to visit his elderly mother in hospital (Blake 2010). A warden in Sandwell in the West Midlands administered a £75 fixed penalty notice to a mother and child feeding bread to ducks (Sharpe 2010). Whilst we do not make claims for the representativeness of these examples, what we can deduce from these kind of incidents is the extent to which penalties are ready to hand for a variety of officials, and how they are also readily relied upon by legislators and policymakers as a means of giving force to policy. In addition, the sheer volume of legislation in the contemporary era has necessitated the dispersal of penality away from the traditional centres of justice in the courts and towards a variety of public employees who did not hitherto have a formally punitive role.

The 1997–2010 New Labour administration pursued a vigorous legislative programme introducing, among other things, nineteen criminal justice acts and the creation of 4,300 new offences (*Daily Telegraph* 2010b). Some of the provisions have not yet been used, such as the ability of the police to specify alcohol disorder zones where licensed premises in troubled areas can be made to contribute towards the costs. Other provisions have been used in a very limited fashion. Since 2005 only 160 penalty notices have been issued for serving alcohol to a drunk person (Slack 2010). Nevertheless, despite the relative infrequency with which some provisions are used, their availability to be activated not only by the police but a variety of other officials means that these representatives themselves have an expanded range of opportunities to embark the citizen upon a course which, whilst it may not be criminal in the first instance, can rapidly lead to criminal sanction.

Prior to this chapter, in discussing the kinds of changes that have taken place in the social policy landscape we have considered those that seem to be in the Foucaldian tradition of 'care of the self' and to foster particular kinds of consciousness, with an emphasis on self-aware self-regulation to enhance independence, entrepreneurialism and responsibility. Yet with the meteoric expansion of legislation under which citizens can be typified as suspects or offenders it is clear that action at a distance and the internalization of the disciplinary gaze is not the whole story where new disciplinary forms of citizenship are afforded. There is a much wider deployment of legislation to observe, coerce and regulate the citizen and the kinds of activities and associations in which he or she might be involved.

There have been a number of attempts to offer an assessment and critique of the legislation that has been introduced in the last couple of decades, especially under the New Labour administration (1997–2010). In a number of popular books – often written from the point of view of little Englander libertarianism – authors have railed against the punitive regulation of everyday life.

For example, Philip Johnston (2010) in *Bad Laws* outlines some of the legislation – which was often based on notions of risk management – that has sought to impose order where otherwise unregulated social life was concerned. The New Labour administration specialized in creating legislation with very broad brush strokes so that it could be applied to a variety of activities which were hitherto relatively lightly regulated. The Terrorism Act 2000 included a wide definition of terrorism so as to enable its use to prohibit political demonstrations; the 2001 Race Relations Act mandated an obligation for schools to report 'racist incidents', including name calling. The Criminal Justice and Police Act 2001 created zones in which the police and community support officers could confiscate bottles of wine from picnickers and also made it an offence to protest outside somebody's home. Under the Sexual Offences Act of 2003 it is potentially an offence to get someone drunk. This Act also criminalized teenagers embracing and kissing. Under the Anti-Social Behaviour Act of 2003, dispersal zones were created in which the police could enforce the break-up of groups of people who had assembled and enabled the imposition of on the spot fines for graffiti, litter, noise and truancy. The Licensing Act of 2003 enabled the regulation of entertainments such as comedians, poetry readings and music in pubs. The Hunting Act 2004 banned fox hunting with dogs and the Health Act 2006 banned smoking in many public places. These pieces of legislation, says Johnston (2010) are largely disconnected from the desires or needs of the public. This regulation is just as likely to be used against the public as on its behalf. Rather, it embodies the worldview of the bureaucratic elite. Much of this legislation is not concerned with seeking a public benefit but merely reflects a particular kind of bureaucratic worldview that is concerned to regulate for its own sake.

As Ross Clark (2006) notes in *How to Label a Goat*, a great deal of the legislation passed is not in the form of Acts of Parliament, subject to debate and a vote. Much of it instead takes the form of statutory instruments. Consequently, parliamentarians have very little scrutiny over it. Promises to reduce regulation and legislation are generally followed up with further legislation instead. Michael Heseltine, on behalf of the previous Conservative government, promised a bonfire of red tape yet this yielded little but rule changes enabling the government of the day to proceed with road building schemes despite local opposition. The New Labour government's Legislative and Regulatory Reform Act (2006) was created ostensibly to enable the simplification of complex or outdated regulations, but instead abrogated to ministers considerable new powers to amend legislation. 'In other words', says Clark (2006, 228), 'the red tape which it wanted to tackle in reality consisted of the parliamentary regulations preventing governments introducing laws at whim'.

Brian Monteith (2009) in *The Bully State* argues that one of the characteristics of policy in the contemporary era is that the state seeks not just to intervene in its citizens' conduct in terms of guidance, but in terms of criminal sanction, loss of livelihood and other severe penalties too. In the last couple of decades there have been a variety of means whereby citizens can be compelled towards the kind of behaviour deemed desirable and the actions deemed undesirable can be more readily subject to sanction without the burden of proof that was required in the past.

Ramsay (2009) places these attempts to control the citizen in relation to what he sees as three broader political trends. These comprise the 'third way', communitarianism and neoliberalism. Giddens's third way recognizes that contemporary society is marked 'by a new individualism in which self-fulfilment is the central object of people's lives' (Ramsay 2009, 135). All three political trends adhere to a notion of so-called 'vulnerable autonomy'. He explains that 'the protection of "vulnerable autonomy" is a norm at the heart of the three political theories with a preponderant influence in contemporary politics in the UK' (Ramsay 2009, 114). Ontological security is a pre-requisite for the achievement of self-fulfilment; this requires the cooperation of others as self-realization 'is always vulnerable to the hostility or indifference of others' (Ramsay 2008, 16).

The idea that citizens as a whole are vulnerable underlies the rationale for the use of restrictive and punitive sanctions for so-called anti-social behaviour. In this view, autonomy among ordinary citizens is seen as dependent on a process of mutual recognition and mutual positive regard. These, however, are

> more or less fragile achievements, and their vulnerability to various forms of injury, violation, and denigration makes it a central matter of justice that the social contexts within which they emerge be protected. (Anderson and Honneth 2005, 137)

In order for the autonomy of citizens to be protected, they must be guaranteed a supportive 'recognitional environment':

> Autonomy turns out to have as a condition of its possibility, a supportive recognitional infrastructure. Because agents are largely dependent on this recognitional infrastructure for their autonomy, they are subject to autonomy-related vulnerabilities: harms to and neglect of these relations of recognition jeopardise individuals' autonomy. (Anderson and Honneth 2005, 145)

Or as the then UK prime minister Tony Blair stated in a debate with Henry Porter in the *Observer*:

> If the practical effect of the law is that people live in fear because the offender is unafraid of the legal process then, in the name of civil liberties, we are allowing the vulnerable, the decent, the people who show respect and expect it back, to have their essential liberties trampled on. (Porter and Blair 2006, 20)

As Giddens (1991, 1998) has documented, in late modernity the autonomy of each individual is seen as dependent on the lifestyle choices of others, entailing a new 'life politics' or politics of lifestyle. This also entails the re-framing of the welfare state as a positive welfare society

> in which welfare is understood as a psychic rather than an economic concept. A positive welfare society is concerned to ensure social cohesion, which is to say cohesion between the different and diverse conditions of the psychic welfare of its self-fulfilling subjects. (Ramsay 2009, 137)

Thus, once the liberties of the individual citizen, his or her autonomy and their ability to go about their lives are framed in this way, the stage is set for punitive intervention in the lives of others who get in their way. The litter louts, nuisance teenagers and persistent petty offenders, those who might have suggestive unsupervised conversations with children and so on, are now identifiable hazards to the civil polity. This then provides the rationale for means to control them and for the lower standards of proof frequently required.

The New Labour administration introduced a variety of means under its legislative programme that could be used in attempts to control the problematic individual's behaviour. Ramsay (2008) points out that a many of these legislative tools that he calls (following Shute 2004) 'civil prevention orders', such as ASBOs, Terrorism Control Orders and Risk of Sexual Harm Orders, share a number of common features such as their being granted in civil proceedings, being granted so as to cover vague and often widely defined behaviour and breach of the terms of the order leading to criminal sanction.

Ramsay (2008, 6) quotes the relevant sections of the Crime and Disorder Act 1998 which govern the granting of ASBO:

(a) that the person has acted...in an anti-social manner, that is to say, in a manner that caused or was likely to cause harassment, alarm or distress to one or more persons not of the same household as himself; and
(b) that such an order is necessary to protect relevant persons from further anti-social acts by him.

In other words, says Ramsay, what these kinds of orders address is the problem of recalcitrant citizens 'manifesting of a disposition of indifference or hostility, a lack of respect for others' feelings' and it is this which 'unifies the conduct which attracts liability to an ASBO' (2008, 7). Civil prevention orders 'share a common substantive content – a liability for a failure to reassure' (Ramsay 2009, 114).

As the Home Office implied in 'Respect and Responsibility' (Home Office 2003, 13), the average citizen is seen as intrinsically vulnerable and it is as if they need reassurance before they will be willing to go about their normal lives. The 'right to be free from harassment, alarm or distress', asserted by the home secretary in the foreword to that document, is the governmental response in order to protect this perceived vulnerability.

The notion that everyday life is poised on a knife edge and is not robust in the face of inconveniences and insults is one of the key justifications for the intensive legislative programme which has been implemented since 1997. Unlike the 'broken windows' approach which typified certain sorts of people – the poor, the drunk and the destitute – as problematic, the contemporary approach identifies much larger swathes of the population as falling within its ambit. Potentially the entire citizenry could fall foul of the legislation as it might be interpreted by zealous officials.

Surveillance is arguably more intensive than in previous eras, both in terms of the technology that can be employed and the opportunities for a variety of official bodies to make use of the information collected and to use covert surveillance techniques. For example, local authorities have used the Regulation of Investigatory Powers Act (RIPA) to investigate whether applicants for a particular popular school do indeed live in its catchment area (Shepherd 2010). Indeed, local authorities are particularly enamoured of the powers they can activate under RIPA, having used them to investigate citizens' conduct in more than 8,500 cases over the two years prior to 2010 according to press reports regarding this issue (Travis 2010). This has included investigations to detect whether people are leaving clothes outside charity shops, identify those whose dogs foul the footpath and to monitor compliance with smoking bans. Local authority employees themselves are examined in a similar manner with RIPA provisions being employed to monitor car parking, the working hours they observe, the activities of those claiming to be off work sick and the job performance of wardens 'employed to spot crime' (Travis 2010, 9).

This is taken by many critics to indicate the advance of the surveillance society and the database state. Certainly the UK is one of the leading nations where the deployment of this kind of technology is concerned. But what is interesting from our point of view is what this means for citizens themselves who might reasonably come to expect that officials are observing them (at least judging by what they will read in the press) and who might suspect that their conduct is under scrutiny with a view to identifying them as miscreants and imposing penalties.

An apparent mistake in a student's examination paper was recently reported in the *Times Higher Education*: 'The UK birth rate is currently increasing. We have more than 700,000 new suspects every year' (Attwood 2010, 12). Despite being presented as a mistake this seems a curiously insightful summary of the situation. The climate of surveillance and suspicion backed up by an enhanced range of legal sanctions drives divisions between groups of people such that it is hard not to see individuals as suspects. The suspicion is fostered between groups in workplaces, between the young and the old, between different groups and interest segments, between worker and manager, parent and child. Trust, whose purported deficiency was the lament of a number of writers whose work we reviewed in the previous chapter, is difficult to reconstruct in these circumstances. Nor is it very hopeful that the sheer magnitude of legislative coercion can be obviated by trust alone, especially when this is urged on citizens and not upon the state and its agencies. The *modus vivendi* between citizen and state has been reshaped as one of observation and coercion rather than trust or consensus. The 'law abiding' citizen is so fragile that a plethora of measures are necessary to protect them. Equally, the citizen's sense of being in a relationship with others is so frail that it is only through the application of a penal matrix of impositions that they can be made to desist from anti-social behaviour.

One of the most interesting effects of this cocktail of surveillance, intrusion and impending penalty on the people subject to it is that of acceptance. The imposition of this new discipline of civil orders is not entirely unwelcome. In cases where a court has ordered a course of action for the defendants, some of the people who have actually been subject to them do not necessarily find the process unsavoury. Positive responses to anti-social behaviour initiatives are not limited to those who could be considered the obvious beneficiaries, such as neighbours, officials or schoolteachers. As Carr (2010) documents, there is a growing body of research evidence indicating that parents required by the courts to attend parenting courses consider them to have been successful (Ghate and Ramella 2002). In addition, says Carr, Dillane, Hill et al.'s (2001) account of the Dundee Families Project reported positive evaluations. This project involved 'problem' families being placed at risk of eviction because of their anti-social behaviour, placed them under intensive surveillance and implemented a robust programme of interventions with the aim of enabling them to sustain a social housing tenancy without incurring complaint from neighbours or officials. The report on the project included positive reports from the parents who had been subject to these interventions (Dillane, Hill et al. 2001). This finding was not an isolated case. Nixon, Hunter et al. (2006) reported on a number of other 'intensive family support projects' or 'family intervention projects' as such interventions are termed. Among the service users who had been subject to these interventions and felt able to comment on the provision, a majority of those interviewed viewed them as overwhelmingly positive.

This demonstrates a curious continuity between the more overtly disciplinary processes of compulsion and the threat of sanctions such as losing one's home and the idea from the people subject to these orders and interventions that they are valuable. Of course, where evaluations are carried out in such a way as to appear integral to the programme, it may be that participants give favourable evaluations in the hope of securing more favourable outcomes for themselves. But the processes at stake here probably go deeper than this. The incorporation of people with multiple problems and vulnerabilities into programmes of this kind represents a process of clientizing the recipient and configuring them as persons in need of intervention and guidance, so that this is how they come to understand themselves. This makes the likelihood of them evaluating any kind of intervention favourably considerably more likely, as they come to understand themselves as subjects who need 'intervention' and the absence of intervention as somehow akin to deprivation or neglect.

Housing Responsibility: Social Housing as a Moral Arena

The study of housing and housing policy has recently seen a number of scholars draw on notions of governmentality and power to explain some of the developments in the organization of social or public housing and in neighbourhood management more generally. In the UK, at the turn of the century the Department of the Environment, Transport and the Regions (DETR) wrote that:

> Our vision of social housing in the 21st Century is one of homes that support balanced, thriving communities and a high quality of life... We want provision that is wide-ranging and customer-focused, and where tenants have real choice and control over their housing. (DETR 2000, 17)

And as McKee (2011, 6) says, policy was infused with notions of active citizens empowered to 'take responsibility'. Choice was to be increased through the transfer of municipal housing stock to social landlords, tenants were to be empowered to become involved in the management of the housing and there was to be enhanced devolution of responsibility for the organization of housing provision to local communities. As McKee remarks, this is as much about the reconstruction of the citizen as it is about the construction of new rationalities of management for housing itself. These policy manoeuvres have gone hand in hand with initiatives such as choice based lettings, good neighbour agreements, family intervention projects and tenant participation (Bradley 2008; Cowan and McDermont 2006; Flint 2003, 2004; McIntyre and McKee 2008; Parr, 2009). This has proceeded on a variety of fronts. For example, under the terms of transfer agreements for housing stock, tenants have been appointed to committees charged with the management of social housing (Bradley 2011), a degree of marketization and 'consumer focus' has been urged upon social housing providers (Pawson and Smith 2009) and tenants have been enlisted in a process of mobilizing and shaping their active involvement in the housing process (McKee and Cooper 2008). These processes have highlighted for many authors the way in which the governmental agenda sometimes has limited power to entirely reshape the tenant. Bradley (2011) documents the friction between tenants and professional managers on committees and boards to manage social housing, noting the exasperation of the latter that tenant representatives insisted on bringing up 'estate level issues' in committee meetings.

For the purposes of this chapter however, we will focus on the more overtly disciplinary projects in social housing policy and practice. Certainly, housing is a tool of policy addressed to making desirable kinds of community and citizens flourish. Yet at the same time, there are some important corollaries of this process of clientizing and disciplining the citizen that we mentioned earlier which can be found directed toward the resident of social housing. It is implicit in many schemes addressed to the tenants of social housing that those who fail to satisfy the conditions of their occupation are somehow morally irresponsible, that is personally culpable for their failure to take responsibility for their conduct and as such it is supposed that they have rendered themselves undeserving of the benefit of occupation within the sector (Cobb 2006, 239). Yau (2011) documents a variety of measures in different nations, from ASBOs in Britain, misconduct-related evictions in the US, through to penalty points for social housing residents in Hong Kong, that may cumulatively jeopardize their tenancies.

Under these kinds of disciplinary frameworks the production of normalization, is not merely a matter of socializing the citizen to afford the growth of responsibility. Instead, it frequently involves directly bringing citizens and their conduct within an expanded grid of control, especially through the marketization of their affective capacities (Clough 2004, 14–15; Willse 2010). Fear, anxiety and vulnerability yield a particularly heady mixture:

> The projection of hate and fear onto a population that makes it into a mythical adversary, may come to function as a support of evaluations of populations, marking some for death and others for life. (Clough 2008, 18)

In Britain, the marginalization of social housing tenants judged to be anti-social was taken forward by a 2011 consultation document proposing the wider use of probationary tenancies, extended powers for social landlords to evict problematic tenants and a range of 'incentives for tenants to behave in a way that respects their neighbours' (Department for Communities and Local Government 2011). The progressive 'othering' of people who are poor, marginalized or rely on social housing has proceeded along with an expansion of the discourse of personal responsibility, and this has been accompanied by the intensification of social welfare technologies that seek to 'regulate the poor' by intervening in individual behaviour (Piven and Cloward [1971] 1993; Willse 2010).

Where the insecurely or socially housed are concerned the motivation toward more intensive regulation is deepened, for as Cobb (2006) notes, governments in the UK continue to frame anti-social behaviour as a problem occurring predominantly in conjunction with social housing, and this means that social landlords are expected to play a role in its control. Under section 218A of the Housing Act 1996, they are obliged to formulate policies for its reduction. Their powers to act are, at the time of writing, to be enhanced in the Localism Bill (Department for Communities and Local Government 2011).

This has led to a process akin to the notion of medicalization that we discussed in the previous chapter. The problematization of housing insecurity and deprivation as if it represented an individual pathology or deficiency opens up the space for disciplinary interventions, especially those modelled on case management technologies. In case management systems, a case worker or social worker assumes authority for guiding the client, or case, through a process of self-evaluation. This often seeks to identify the 'needs' or individual causes underlying their problem. Worker and client then develop a case plan or care plan which, whilst it may ostensibly involve collaboration and a process of working together, may well involve an element of compulsion and operate within the confines of non-negotiable programme requirements (Willse 2010). Such plans might involve participation in educational, vocational or drug rehabilitation programmes and instruction in money management and 'employability' skills. Thus, according to Willse (2010, 165), with the development of a professional class of social workers and related occupations, 'the idea of "working on yourself" as a necessary part of securing and maintaining housing was routinized and codified in technologies of case management'. It is this process of seeing the insecurely housed self as being in need of remediation and case management that have prompted scholars like Willse (2010) to identify what they see as being a kind of 'medicalization of homelessness'. Thus, difficulties with housing, failure to remain housed, housing deprivation and even frequent moves of home may be treated as a symptom of personal pathology that must be cured by experts (Cress and Snow 2000; Lyon-Callo 2004). Whilst eviction may be a last resort, there may be, as a precursor to this, a variety of ways in which problematic tenants are enjoined to work upon themselves to 'address' the problem.

Where housing is concerned, programmes to address homelessness, problem tenants, neighbours from hell and insecurely housed individuals are increasingly seen as part of the neoliberal governmentality project (McKee 2011) and therefore facilitate the very conditions and systems that produce housing insecurity and deprivation. This in turn is part of what Wacquant (2008, 9) describes as 'social polarisation and punitive upsurge'. Plans to address homelessness, problem families and the like often come into being through the endorsement of national and local government, the police and business lobby groups keen to support any effort to remove unsheltered, uncivil or unsightly individuals from public view. Rather like the focus of Wilson and Kelling's 'broken windows', the focus is not primarily on the infrastructure or the windows themselves, but rather on the human element that accompanies them. In this sense, plans and policies surrounding housing activate and sustain a medicalized conception of housing problems where the unhoused or problem tenants are concerned, as if removing 'problem individuals' from 'the streets' or 'neighbours from hell' from estates is an adequate solution. Despite these remedial efforts, insecure labour markets, fluctuating interest rates, shortages of accommodation, failures to invest in infrastructure, the criminal justice system, prisons, privatized housing and inadequate public assistance programmes will continue to produce unsheltered populations and problem tenants.

Once problem tenants and neighbours from hell have been identified, both public sector and social housing officials are pressed into a reconfigured role of policing the tenants and playing a part in imposing sanction on those who fall short of the criteria of good citizenship. People in need of accommodation are, as we have seen, conceived of as 'moral members of responsible communities' who should be willing and able to refrain from anti-social behaviour (Flint 2003, 615). The leverage employed by housing providers to shape this kind of responsible moral agency is conditionality of housing provision. An individual's entitlement to occupation within the sector is increasingly dependent upon their satisfying provisions of good behaviour and even, in some cases, willingness to engage in approved community processes intended to foster neighbourhood social capital. Housing agencies are increasingly key players in laying out the parameters of officially approved identities for those to be governed, by striving to create solutions to the perceived problem by attempting to foster a constructed image of 'community' (Flint 2003, 2004).

To illustrate how people who live in social housing are constructed as potentially problematic citizens and some of the tensions in the construction of 'community' in such contexts, let us consider another example from rural Wales. We know of one region in which the former council housing stock has been transferred to another social landlord. Much of this housing is made up of properties built in the last century, situated in villages and small towns scattered across a mountain region. Many of the tenants are elderly, having been tenants of the same property for decades. Others are the adult children of earlier tenants, having 'inherited' the tenancy when this was possible. In many cases, the tenants of neighbouring properties, if not actually related to each other, have usually grown up together. The social landlord now responsible for managing these houses sent all tenants a lengthy leaflet describing their responsibilities as tenants and how this involves – as well as paying ones rent and desisting from anti-social behaviour – actively participating in the 'community'; it also recently placed an advert in the situations vacant pages of the local paper for a 'community involvement support officer'.

To anyone familiar with this region, this is extraordinary – this ethnolinguistically cohesive part of Wales has as strong a sense of community as is possible to find in the UK at present. Whilst some of the village communities have identified problems with 'anti-social' behaviour, the nature of this tends to be teenagers gathering around the doorways of the local shops in the evenings, drinking or making much noise. This undoubtedly irritating behaviour is probably more a function of being a bored teenager with little money living in an isolated hill village, than an indication of developing serious criminality. Even in the towns in this region, the most serious identified problems concern people who are severely mentally ill or have addiction problems. Yet many of the residents of this area are now constructed as a potential source of crime, an incipient risk to community cohesion and as being in need of instruction regarding how to be part of a 'community' because they do not own their houses.

Therefore, as Flint has noted, increasingly social housing agencies in the UK in their role as governing bodies purport to be able to specify what constitutes good, appropriate and responsible conduct (Dean 1999) and seek to direct the actions of their tenants. This may involve housing bodies in attempts to address anti-social behaviour by encouraging self-regulation and responsibility amongst their tenants. This proactive and often moralizing stance attempts to shape acceptable behaviour in relation to other residents and broader responsibilities towards 'the community'. Flint (2003) suggests that this explicit moral dimension is distinctive to British social policy, particularly where social housing is concerned (Haworth and Manzi 1999). With press reports in the UK indicating that there may be as many as 5,000,000 people on social housing waiting lists (Kollewe 2010), it is increasingly possible for social housing agencies to be selective in terms of who they house. Under recent coalition government proposals, social housing agencies will have increased powers to refuse tenants who fall behind with rent (Ramesh and Wintour 2010). Therefore, social housing agencies in the UK are in a stronger position to attempt to define the 'responsible' behaviour demanded of their tenants. This is enhanced under current coalition government proposals to introduce time limited and means tested tenancies for local authority accommodation. In this way, opportunities have been extended for enforcing standards of behaviour which purport to reflect the commonly held values of 'the community' and which emphasize residents' responsibilities to conduct themselves so as not to impair the amenity of their neighbours of such a community. Failures of the individual to comply with the standards that accompany the tenancy, or that might be imposed by any schemes in which they are enrolled, may enable social housing agencies to exert a more explicit disciplinary power over tenants.

Within housing policy as a whole, the anti-social tenant is viewed as a risk not only to the quality of life of individual residents but to the reputation of entire estates or neighbourhoods and the possibility that the area will become, or remain, 'difficult to let' (Cobb 2006, 244). Therefore, the disciplinary measures applied to tenants who might fall short of the standards demanded – even though they might represent a small minority – are themselves an important aspect of wider housing strategies. Whilst being subject to the threat of losing their home and to a variety of what Ramsay (2009) calls civil enforcement orders, the problem tenant and the schemes to bring them under control is part of a broader process of maintaining gradients of desirability in housing stock and residential areas themselves. Problem tenants have an iconic value in terms of maintaining differentiation between desirable areas and those deemed to be 'sink estates', with a corresponding financial premium on the areas deemed more salubrious. Better amenities, schools with more coveted places in league tables and a variety of reductions in morbidity and mortality attach to the neighbourhoods where accommodation is more expensive. These divisions and gradients of differentiation are crucial in maintaining value in the housing stock. If problem tenants did not exist perhaps they would need to be invented.

Quis Custodiet Ipsos Custodes?: Disciplining the Professionals

The pattern of scrutiny and the availability of coercive sanction is not confined to those at the very bottom of the hierarchy of wealth, status and prestige. As we have seen, the proliferation of the grid of possible sanctions means that everyone is a potential suspect and potentially anyone can be subject to penalty or sanction. It will come as no surprise then that the public servants who implement these regimes themselves are subject to quality assurance procedures, audit and review. If they are sufficiently junior, a range of sanctions can be employed if they are found wanting. Thus, a mechanical model of rules and punishments is unfolded throughout the career course in both public and private life. Meeting targets, obeying rules and seeking to maintain the self as a functional economic unit of production (and perhaps more importantly consumption) is undertaken through increasingly complex and capricious disciplinary grids.

In coming to an understanding of how surveillance of the professions had risen to such prominence under advanced liberalism and how it is replacing trust, Brown and Calnan (2009) turn to the work of Richard Sennett on what he calls 'craftsmanship'. Sennett (2008, 6) argues that work has the potential to become an end in itself to the extent that the overarching effects of the craft come to be of secondary importance. Work may take on a value in its own right, independently of its benefits or pitfalls as they might appear to an outsider. As Brown and Calnan (2009) argue much as the craftsman may lose him or herself in the work so that 'nothing else matters' (Sennett 2008, 6), so too may notions of the human ambitions of a public service become lost in the midst of bureaucracy to audit, manage and measure it, to the extent that only 'convention, efficiency and "internal coherence"' (Marcuse 1989, 121) come to be of significance.

Allied to the renewed vitality of audit, measurement and targets has been the reformulation of organized social life in terms of risks and their regulation. Rothstein (2006) argues that the internal logic of risk regulation means that what is minimized is risk posed towards the institution, rather than towards the individuals served by this institution. Risk and risk minimization appear to be unassailable arguments. Who, after all, could argue that risk should be increased? Especially where likelihoods are expressed numerically, this gives a sense of precision to the potential for success and failure in attempting to manage the problems that the institution faces. The more effectively and precisely such governance is carried out, the more sensitive institutions become towards the prospect of failing to successfully manage risks: '"good governance" gives rise to risk itself' (Rothstein 2006, 217). Under the auspices of managing risk, a great many social issues have become reformulated as issues of risk. This enables the institutions responsible to address the accountability and liability of their decision making in response to audit inspection or litigation, but whether practice and service delivery are improved remains a moot point. Where procedures and guidelines are followed there may be large swathes of practice and many client problems that the organization simply does not have the capacity or agility to address.

The drift of government policy over the last two decades has been toward greater use of audit and targets as ways of managing and enhancing performance. Yet, as a growing literature shows, both in theory (Gallivan and Depledge 2003; Bevan and Hood 2006) and in practice (Public Administration Select Committee 2003; Som 2005) the inspections and auditing by public bodies and the regularly announced 'challenging new targets' are limited in their effectiveness in assuring compliance and therefore performance. This is particularly so where the services and processes themselves have been wholly or partially privatized and outsourced, so the effective reach of control is symbolic rather than practical. Employees charged with managing service delivery may have relatively little effective control despite what may be promised in policy documents (Crawford and Brown 2008). As Brown and Calnan (2009) argue, the likelihood that control mechanisms will be undermined is increased where new frameworks are seen to compromise the craftsmanship or artistry of the human service professionals involved. In the case of medicine, the resistance to a culture of oversight has been noticeable (Brown 2008), as it is the professional knowledge and the craft aspects of the work which give meaning to practitioners' actions and the associated meaning, values and norms that govern individuals' actions (Habermas 1987).

Even when it is not readily possible to detect what meaning the rules, protocols and manuals have, this does not necessarily compromise their power to compel compliance. The bureaucratic burden necessitates and compels a 'blind self-preservation' (Habermas 1984, 398) that will ensure at least superficial compliance within these bureaucratic stipulations and measures.

But there is more to these policies that insist on repeated inspection, perpetual monitoring, ongoing surveillance and requirements for continual revalidation. They also demonstrate a lack of trust in the practitioners whose performance is the subject of inspection and review. The burden of encouraging and verifying good craftsmanship and economic efficiency further erodes trust between managers and professionals, professionals and clients and amongst professionals themselves (Calnan and Rowe 2008). A moment's reflection on the time and energy expended on the examination, audit and inspection processes will suffice to apprehend just how enormous this burden can become and how it can be a distraction away from the client or service user. In the case of hospital treatment for example, prospective patients may have information that gives them greater choice and the opportunity to avoid institutional risks and poor performance. This does not necessarily result in their gaining an enhanced experience of healthcare, because their individual experience is profoundly shaped by the kind of communicative relationship that they enjoy with health professionals and ancillary staff (Brown 2008). Their experience may be compromised by choice, especially where 'choice becomes a "new paternalism" in which the availability of a patient-centred service, a high priority for users, does not figure on the agenda of providers' (Taylor-Gooby 2008, 165).

Conclusion

This brief survey of the variegated forms of coercion and potential for penalty which is immanent across a number of areas of contemporary social life has attempted to show how the process has developed in policy and in practice and how it contributes to the disciplinary project of responsibilization. Anti-social behaviour initiatives, especially those which mandate involvement of the targeted individual in classes, curfews and contracts, represent a distinctive governmental response to the inherent insecurity of advanced liberalism and the 'vulnerable autonomy' of the citizen, which may be threatened by conduct which is uncivil or disorderly. As well as being integral to New Labour's 'Third Way' policies, these look set to continue in large measure under the coalition government. For Carr (2010), they go hand in hand with the inability of government to reassure its citizens that it can protect them from global insecurities, austerity and the effects of global movements of capital. Instead, the responsibility to reassure one another is cast upon the citizens themselves, as they are mandated not to threaten, annoy or otherwise discommode one another, lest a penalty or civil prevention order be applied.

Theresa Funiciello (1993) describes the service model of welfare provision as a 'tyranny of kindness'. That is, welfare programmes designed to address housing difficulties, parenting deficiencies, disorder and anti-social behaviour frequently signal the paternalistic and coercive nature of the interventions concerned, often demanding submission to reform protocols in the name of the client's own good. Funiciello's term therefore gets to the heart of the tension in disciplinary power as described by Foucault. Ostensibly humanistic projects intended to develop mental and physical capacities – and responsibility itself – often proceed through mechanisms of submission and control. Thus, policymakers and human service professionals may be found proceeding through regimes of submission in order to improve and liberate the citizen (Foucault [1975] 1995). In order to preserve their entitlement to social welfare, affordable housing or freedom itself, individuals have to show that they meet certain conditions (Deacon 2004; Dwyer 2004; Taylor-Gooby 2005). This welfare conditionality means that with acts of provision such as welfare benefits or housing, come obligations and conditions for the recipient. Governable citizens are, in an important sense, 'subjects of doubt' (Clarke 2004). They may be capable not only of resisting the attempts of managers and policymakers to regulate their behaviour, but may also be involved in creating their own governmental strategies, either in partnership with, or against, various authorities. Thus, people who have been subject to civil control orders of various kinds may on the one hand seek to remain uncooperative, or on the other actively work with the intervention and end up saying they found it helpful. Governable subjects are often formulated as needing to be shaped and guided, as well as mobilized, so as to develop personal power and the 'control of one's self' (McKee 2011, 5), perhaps aided by the threat of impending sanctions if they fail to make use of the amenities in an approved manner.

This matrix of discipline is also accompanied by a grid of visibility thrown over the officials and service agents responsible for managing the welfare and health arena, who are subject to audit, inspection and performance management themselves. They are subject to 'a discourse of empowerment and autonomy, implicated within frameworks of increasing accountability for life' (Flint 2004, 153).

Welfare, civility and responsibility in the social arena then is managed through a complex network of sanctions and penality. Whilst prison has expanded its grasp of the population in many nations, the carceral itself is only able to contain a fraction of the population. Its centrality to economic and civic life, though, means that it casts a long shadow over a variety of other sanctions, even though they may not be criminal matters in the first place. The risks believed to be attendant upon disreputable behaviour help to justify a progressive system of interventions and sanctions to manage civic life.

Chapter Eight

THINKING ABOUT OURSELVES

Introduction: Reflexive Work on the Self

In this chapter, we take a closer look at what all the reflection on the entrepreneurial self-producing and self-projecting self that we described in the previous chapters might mean. The matrix of forces described earlier, with a variety of fields of public service and therapeutic enterprise emphasizing the importance of the individual taking responsibility, encourages a particular kind of consciousness in the early twenty-first century under conditions of advanced liberalism.

The broad spectrum of encouragement toward greater responsibility necessitates an increasingly reflexive kind of work on the self. As a number of commentators such as Giddens (1991) and Beck (1992) have proposed, this is a kind of self which is self-produced as a result of the techniques of biography and through fostering the ability to apprehend and reflect upon the risks that surround the self. For Giddens and Beck this represents a model of the self that can be universally applied. For Beck, whilst individuals are not able to escape structural forces in general, they are to some extent able to decide which forces they should act upon and which can be ignored. This, says Beck, does not create a 'free' individual, but instead yields individuals whose biographies embody or live out the complexity and diversity of the social relations in which they are embedded.

In this chapter we will begin with some reflections on the idea that selves are a kind of project, an idea found especially within the work of Anthony Giddens and Zygmunt Baumann. For these authors, the individual is characterized as a being with profound and overarching needs for meaning and autonomy, apt to assemble a self-image in the manner of a consumer, choosing an assemblage of objects, artefacts and stories. Earlier, pre-modern notions of the place of humanity in a broader cosmological system was challenged by thinkers and activists in the Protestant reformation, and followed up by broader processes of detraditionalization and secularization. Latterly, we have seen the ascendance of authenticity as a key value, and this has gone hand in hand with new secularized forms of confession in the form of therapy, life story telling and personal development. Experience of working life and social relationships may nowadays be fragmented and assembled and reassembled many times over through the life course, so the self-narrative itself assumes a new degree of prominence and significance. The modern self-narrative is often also one of confession through therapy, self-help, reality TV, needs assessments and other processes of self-disclosure. This may, in some cases, involve disclosures about the body as well as the psyche through assemblages of fashion, fascination with celebrities, paternity tests, tests for the presence of sexually transmitted infections and the like, many of which can be found as basic staples of daytime TV. There are even a variety of self-help sources for those seeking to reinvent themselves as a personal brand. But through all this, the image consultants counsel, one needs to preserve the sense of authenticity which is at the core of the self.

It is this self, this biographical production, that is central to what Beck calls 'reflexive modernity'. Giddens sees what he calls 'institutional reflexivity' as fundamental to the development of a new universal 'life politics' in which individuals are concerned to construct a coherent biography in a fractured world. By institutional reflexivity Giddens means that the process whereby the analysis and discussion of society – the way society sees itself – situated in major societal institutions and often conducted by experts, in turn shapes that society. Giddens (1991) envisions institutional reflexivity as a diachronic process – the degree or density of reflexivity increases over time. Under these circumstances, the self becomes a project on which the individual can work reflexively in order to produce some sense of coherence.

From the point of view of social science, it is as if the model of the self is one which owes something to Blumer (1969), in which the self can be regarded as '...a sensitizing concept, a heuristic tool, to orient ourselves and understand the processes that constitute inner life and society' (Rambo 2007, 538). In this way, as well as trying to describe the mechanisms of selfhood and self-construction, it is also a concept that provides a lens for looking at the individual and his or her conduct. The self is seen as a kind of project. This process of creation of the self is described by Thompson (1995, 210):

> It is a project that the individual constructs out of the symbolic materials which are available to him or her, materials which the individual weaves into a coherent account of who he or she is, a narrative of self-identity.

This project of the self is a reflexive one – it is pursued in a self-aware, self-directing manner. As Korsgaard notes: 'When you deliberate, it is as if there were something over and above all of your desires, something which is *you*, and which *chooses* which desire to act on' (1996, 83). There is a curiously out of body experience to this executive part of the self. The strategic direction seems to come from something over and above this self and its corporeal desires and seems distinct from the individual's emotional propensities.

This reflexive project of the self is often seen as being somewhat precarious. We are faced with existential questions about our own identity, when we are confronted with 'personal meaninglessness… a fundamental psychic problem in circumstances of late modernity' (Giddens 1991, 9). This 'looming threat of personal meaninglessness' is a consequence of what Giddens sees to be a 'morally arid social environment' due in partly to 'the pervasiveness of abstract systems' (1991, 201).

Bauman (1989, 189) points out that:

> Individual needs of personal autonomy, self-definition, authentic life or personal perfection are all translated into the need to possess, and consume, market-offered goods. This translation, however, pertains to the appearance of use value of such goods, rather than to the use value itself; as such, it is intrinsically inadequate and ultimately self-defeating, leading to momentary assuagement of desires and lasting frustration of needs.

In the view of several contemporary social theorists, people are assembling their contemporary sense of self from consumption opportunities rather than, for example, community or religion. The contemporary sense of self is a kind of dual self. That is, it involves a self that continually reflects upon itself, separating the self from social relations so that the former can reflect and plan its future actions, yet at the same time reinserting itself back into society through internalization. Thus it is a self that 'knows itself'.

Through scrupulous work on the self, we are enjoined to respond to the risks posed by our environments and our lifestyles. If we exercise and cultivate a positive attitude we are told that this will reduce the risk of heart disease, stroke and even cancer. Marriages, friendships and parent-child relations require incessant expert approved work in order to function. We think about ourselves in terms of the necessity for self-fulfilment, self-improvement and personal development. At the same time, limitations in income and opportunities make this a mirage for all but a small proportion of the population. Selves increasingly come to be defined in terms of the commodities and brands with which they can be associated. The self is a project in which we must continually invest in order to keep pace with a world where the ability to accommodate 'change' is cast as a virtue. To harmonize ourselves with the unstable and fluctuating labour market we must incessantly recreate ourselves through training, updating and education to keep pace with the demands of workplaces within which competition, league tables, performance tables and records of attainment have been meticulously introduced.

The Genealogy of the Modern Self

So convincing is the modern sense of self that, as philosopher Charles Taylor (1988, 299) states, we tend to believe 'we have selves as we have eyes, hearts, or livers'. Yet things have not always been like this. Looking at the broad sweep of history or across the world's different civilizations one can detect other arrangements. As Taylor reminds us, prior to the modern era, Westerners, like many residents in other cultures nowadays, believed in what Taylor (1989) calls a 'two-tiered' vision of the world which as its name suggests, incorporated two key elements. First, there was a broad cosmological framework that provided the world with meaning and value, and second there was an understanding of mundane day to day life that derived meaning from these broader frameworks. Some of these ideas can be seen in late medieval or renaissance concepts – the heavens, the four winds, the ages of man, the signs of the zodiac and so on.

The ascendant view in Western contemporary secular understandings of the human condition however focuses instead only on a single tier. A number of writers (Berger 1977; MacPherson 1962; Richardson 1989; Weber 1978) have suggested that this 'one-tiered' vision of the world emerged in response to a variety of economic, political, social and intellectual movements from the sixteenth to the eighteenth centuries. Events such as the Protestant Reformation, the American and French Revolutions, the political and social turbulence in many nations in the early nineteenth century, the Enlightenment and the scientific revolution, all served to destabilize hierarchies and what we would now consider to be patterns of oppression. The intensely individual focus of the theologies of John Knox (c.1510–1572), George Wishart (1513–1546) and John Calvin (1509–1564) encouraged the questioning of structures of power, authority and inequality inherent in pre-modern hierarchical frameworks. The turbulent relationship between these early Protestants and the contemporary structures of theological and state authority that they opposed helped to embed the single-tiered view, as authority was not to be trusted.

The labour expended against these traditional hierarchies succeeded in collapsing the earlier two-tiered system, in which theological and cosmological frameworks were considered necessary for meaning, into a one-tiered system in which such frameworks were viewed as optional, arbitrary or as somehow metaphysical and at odds with the new scientific world view and the new civil polity that came to prevail, especially after the English Civil War, as the world was increasingly understood in material and mechanical terms.

This change from a two-tiered to a one-tiered framework had major consequences for self-understandings. This is because, as Taylor (1985, 258) claims:

> To define my identity is to define what I must be in contact with in order to function fully as a human agent, and specifically to be able to judge and discriminate and recognize what is really of worth or importance, both in general and for me.

In the old two-tiered system, in order to know what is right to do and good to be, one must be in contact with an external source, such as God, the natural order, the social order, one's family or community. In contrast, from the modern single-tiered point of view 'the horizon of identity is an inner horizon' (Taylor 1985, 258). In this one-tiered system, it is the individual alone who is responsible for determining the nature of the good life, identifying values or determining appropriate courses of action. Often this is, arguably, accomplished through doing nothing more than being one's 'real' self or being authentic (Guignon 2004). Consequently, any attempt to prescribe norms or standards is met with suspicion. Defining virtue, value, happiness or what we might nowadays call 'wellbeing', in terms of some grander reference or standard is often treated as if it were a problem (Christopher and Hickinbottom 2008). The stage is set for a focus on the self as the touchstone of moral authority and touchstone of value.

Consolidating the Single-Tiered World View: Detraditionalization

This process of moving from a two-tiered to a single-tiered system has been further consolidated in recent years by means of a related process that has characterized modernity, termed 'detraditionalization' by a number of commentators. The detraditionalization process has further underpinned the sovereignty of the self and has brought into being a situation where the self can be subject to an accumulated labour of self-investment. Investing in oneself through enhancing one's capacities, undertaking education, taking on responsibilities and the like, becomes not only feasible and legitimate as a thing to do, but also actively encouraged from a variety of sources, from popular self-help literature to government policy.

Let us therefore explore the idea of detraditionalization further, for within it lie some clues about the shaping of the modern self. Traditions, it is claimed, have been dissolved or eroded in many developed societies. But what were traditions exactly? Perhaps if we were to examine what they did, we can see how the social practices and ways of enhancing one's identity that replaced them have become popular. Thompson (1996) identifies four aspects of tradition. These are the 'hermeneutic aspect', the 'normative aspect', the 'legitimation aspect' and the 'identity aspect'. The hermeneutic aspect consists of a body of implicit norms or assumptions that are taken for granted in people's daily lives and are transmitted from one generation to the next. The normative aspect includes the beliefs and patterns of activity that are knowingly taken over from the past. The legitimation aspect involves the means by which power and authority are established and supported. Max Weber, for example, claimed that the legitimacy of a system of domination could be based on belief in the sanctity of traditional authority. The last aspect involves identity formation and how one perceives oneself in a social setting. According to Thompson (1996), there are two types of identity formation. 'Self-identity' is the sense of oneself as an individual, whilst 'collective identity' is a sense of belonging to a particular social group.

Detraditionalization occurs when people stop creating their lives and identities according to social or community context and instead establish their identity based on their individual context. Heelas (1996) suggests that with detraditionalization, people lose their belief in established orders and faith in the values, beliefs or forms of behaviour inherited from tradition is undermined. Detraditionalization involves individuals becoming detached from the cultural contexts to which they once belonged and a shift in authority to the 'individual' through the acquisition of new individualistic values. In late modernity, individuals are charged with making for themselves a lifestyle (Featherstone 1991) and it is increasingly claimed that individuals create and mould their identity or identities (Bauman 1988; Maffesoli 1988; Giddens 1991; Beck 1992) through the symbolic capacities of consumption (Lury 1996) and the acquisition of personal cultural capital. According to this body of thought, 'we have no choice but to choose' (Giddens 1991, 81) because of 'detraditionalization', the weakening of traditional foundations of identity, such as class, the extended family and local settings – all consequences of geographical and social mobility. As Slater (1997, 85) describes, identities are no longer 'unproblematically assigned to us', but understood through the image we create of ourselves through education, occupation, lifestyle or consumption. We choose our self-identity and are required to 'produce and sell an identity to various social markets'.

Under the conditions of neoliberalism and detraditionalization, a sense of personal freedom is fostered, where the self is perceived to have an independent trajectory and self-fulfilment becomes an objective. Gewirth (1998) defined self-fulfilment as an unfolding process comprising two related aspects – aspirations and perceived capabilities. Both aspects combine to delineate primary sources through which a specific individual is likely to find fulfilment. The self could be said to be fulfilled 'when one's deepest aspirations and best capabilities are brought to fruition' (Henry 2006, 171).

Yet this process of self-fulfilment undertaken by the self under conditions of detraditionalization is not necessarily quite as free as it might at first appear. As Marshall and Marshall (1997, 137) warn,

> because they have been constituted to think that they are free and autonomous…this very constitution has permitted the advance of power/ knowledge and the subjugation of people as subjects to lead useful, docile and practical lives.

Self-Examination and Confession

Therefore, the notion of the self is a complex one. Even in this brief sketch of the influences and contexts of the self we can see that there are a number of sometimes contradictory sources. Under these conditions, a humanistic self – a conscious, agentic, stable, unified, bounded, all knowing, rationale, autonomous, ahistorical, present individual (St. Pierre 2000) – is difficult to bring into being simply. The 'I' that we speak about is no longer an obvious and transparent thing – if indeed it ever was. It needs exposing through diligent self-examination, a mystery even to the individual him or herself, something that they are enjoined to dig into their own consciousness to discover

> the particular type of discourse and particular techniques which supposedly reveal our deepest selves…in confession after confession to oneself and to others, this *mise en discourse* has placed the individual in a network of relations of power with those who claim to be able to extract the truth of these confessions through their possession of the keys of interpretations. (Dreyfus and Rabinow 1982, 174)

The kind of self that is encouraged in the contemporary era is a confessional one. Whilst religious confession in the UK has receded in its importance since the Reformation, a variety of other disciplines have risen to take its place. Psychotherapy, whose similarities with confessional activities have been well explored, is the most obvious example. Gellner characterized psychoanalysis as a secularized version of Christianity (Gellner 1993, 37–8). Foucault (1990, 61–2) maintained that 'Western man has become a confessing animal'. Confession is

> also a ritual that unfolds within a power relationship, for one does not confess without the presence (or virtual presence) of a partner who is not simply the interlocutor but the authority who requires the confession, prescribes and appreciates it, and intervenes in order to judge, punish,

forgive, console, and reconcile; a ritual in which the truth is corroborated by the obstacles and resistances it has had to surmount in order to be formulated.

In some cases the confession, especially in the modern era, is freely given and is seen as integral to the process of making sense of ourselves (Wright 2009). Telling the story of one's life has, over the last few decades, gained purchase as a social scientific enterprise. Termed variously life story (McAdams 1997), self-narrative, personal narrative (Richardson 2000; Scheibe 1986) and autobiography, forms of autoethnographic writing (Wright 2009) are accepted as a methodological approach in many academic disciplines (Ellis 2009) and as a therapeutic resource (Grant 2010; Ronai 1995). An academic industry has grown up around life story writing and the methodological and ethical issues it invites. This yields additional layers of self-disclosure and self-scrutiny (Jago 2011; Tolich 2009). The lives of the researchers are often played out as if they were situation comedies or soap operas in the pages of journals dealing with ethnography or qualitative inquiry. There is, at the same time, surprisingly little critical interrogation of the conventionalized motifs and narrative devices that are used to characterize family life. Relationships with step children, overcoming childhood abuse or surviving alcohol problems are all played out as if they were an episode of popular drama or a confessional television show, with little interrogation of the broader system of values that makes these incidents problematic in the first place, or the narrative conventions that give them shape and form.

There is a growing discussion of the ethics of autoethnography. The life story is often a joint production, inasmuch as the writer discloses much detail about other people, often therapists, spouses, sons, daughters, parents or work colleagues. To what extent is the writer bound to seek informed consent from these people? (Tolich 2009). Aside from its effects on the rights of the people mentioned in autoethnographies, this sort of discussion has other effects. The discussion makes writing of this kind seem more real. It is as if the writer is providing something more than the work of a casual autobiographer, writer of memoirs or journalist. These impressions are so real, their description so veridical, the details so intimate, that the writer is somehow breaking the trust of the people who are being written about. There are other ways of seeing memories and autobiographies, of course, but by engaging in these debates these commentators on autoethnography are making it out to be an intimate veridical record.

As a counter to this literalness, one could take the view that in a fundamental and continual way in which we invent or 'fictionalize' ourselves, a 'fictional distance' opens up between the account and the flesh and blood individuals on whom it might be based. It is no wonder that Olney (1980, 92) highlights 'an anxiety about the self, an anxiety about the dimness and vulnerability of that entity that no one has ever seen or touched or tasted'. Like the film-maker Bunuel, we might only speak of autobiographical memory as 'wholly mine – with my affirmations, my hesitations, my repetitions and lapses, my truth and my lies' (Conway 1990, 10). Indeed, as the English Romantic poet John Clare did, we might consider biography to be a total 'pack of lies' (Foss and Trick 1989).

Yet the incorporation of the writer's own story into the ethnographic mix is beset with no such uncertainty. They and the people around them are literally and unproblematically there, untroubled by any postmodern concerns about the fragmentation of identity or any constructionist axioms about social reality being fabricated in situ. Who we are, what has happened to us and our biographical trajectory are coterminous with the truth and authenticity of the self.

Even where there is no intended audience, the storytelling process is believed to have truth-telling powers:

> Confessional writing in diaries was acceptable in our family because it was writing that was never meant to be read by anyone. Keeping a daily diary did not mean that I was seriously called to write, that I would ever write for a reading public. This was 'safe' writing…I could be angry there with no threat of punishment. I could 'talk back.' Nothing had to be concealed. I could hold on to myself there. (hooks 1999, 4–5)

Or as Giddens put it:

> A person's identity is not to be found in behaviour nor – important though this is – in the reactions of others, but in the capacity to keep a particular narrative going. (1991, 54)

In this way perhaps we can begin to formulate an answer to the question that Richard Sennett posed rhetorically:

> How can a human being develop a narrative of identity and life history in a society composed of episodes and fragments? The conditions of the new economy feed instead on experience which drifts in time, from place to place, from job to job… (Sennett 1998, 26)

The key then is confession. In a sense, we confess ourselves into being from the fragments of experience, cultural commonplaces and identity resources at our disposal. The project to maintain our identities is aided by the symbolic resources at our disposal (Sarup 1996). Literature, advertising, brands, television soap operas, music and romantic fiction are all examples of some of the symbolic resources that people draw on and have formed the basis for a number of studies (Radway 1984; Ang 1985; O'Donohoe 1994; Goulding, Shankar et al. 2002; Elliott and Wattanasuwan 1998).

Self-creation and self-fulfilment, whilst they are often discussed as if they were part of a natural emergence of who we 'really are', often rely on a highly specific set of practices through which they are cultivated. These deployments of techniques and practices – or 'technologies of the self' – are in our view central to the production of the self under advanced liberalism. Following Foucault, we understand technologies of the self as a panoply of techniques through which people can work upon or change themselves. In classical antiquity, stoic philosophers advocated a kind of stocktaking of the self. In medieval Christianity, the notion that thoughts as well as deeds could lead to punishment in the hereafter encouraged introspection and confession, and notions of the self and consciousness developed by leaps and bounds. Technologies of the self that define the individual and enable him or her to control their own conduct (Marshall 1996; Besley 2005) have characterized modernity.

Foucault (1985, 29) in *The Use of Pleasure* describes technologies of the self as follows: they are 'models proposed for setting up and developing relationships with the self, for self-reflection, self-knowledge, self-examination, for deciphering the self by oneself, for the transformation one seeks to accomplish with oneself as object'. The notion of confession is central to the new, post-traditional, single-tiered, privatized individual. According to Foucault, confessional culture assumed that a 'principle of latency' is inherent to the individual's conduct (1990, 66). In other words, latency meant there was a 'labour of confession' in which the person making the confession had to be pushed and prodded to understand and reveal the truths about their soul. The embedded and intertwined social relationships that undergirded the 'traditional' or two-tiered version of the world are progressively replaced by a one to one confessional process urged upon the citizen.

We can see this at work in a variety of contexts. The individual's responsibility to take charge of their wellbeing and beat 'stress', for example, is urged partly through a latter day process of confession. An NHS web page tells us how to do so, embellished with advice from 'stress expert' Professor Cary Cooper:

A problem shared is a problem halved, as the old saying goes. A good support network of colleagues, friends and family can ease your work troubles and help you see things in a different way.

'If you don't connect with people, you won't have support to turn to when you need help,' says Professor Cooper. The activities we do with friends help us relax and we often have a good laugh with them, which is an excellent stress reliever.

'Talking things through with a friend will also help you find solutions to your problems,' says Professor Cooper. (NHS 2011)

This is just one example of the myriad ways in which the citizen is enjoined to talk, disclose and confess, the value of which is underscored by appeals to expertise. The labour of confession is supplemented by expert advice as to its beneficence and, as above, is often accompanied by meticulously crafted instructions as to how and to whom these disclosures should be made. As Foucault presciently put it:

> Western societies have established the confession as one of the main rituals we rely on for the production of truth...confessional techniques... the development of methods of interrogation and inquest...the setting up of tribunals of Inquisition: all this helped to give the confession a central role in the order of civil and religious powers... The confession became one of the West's most highly valued techniques for producing truth. We have since become a singularly confessing society. (Foucault 1990, 58–9)

Confession takes place in intimate relationships, in friendships and between work colleagues, as well as in a variety of public fora. As well as the appearances made by supposedly ordinary people and their tragedies in popular magazines, the confession can extend to participation in television programming too. In the UK, the popular daytime television audience discussion programme the *Jeremy Kyle Show* (22 November 2010) invited guests to undertake tests for sexually transmitted infections, the results of which were disclosed to them on air. The show also regularly submits guests to DNA tests to determine the paternity of children. As well as the verbal disclosures which have been the staple of a variety of television shows – usually named eponymously after their host – in this case the disclosures are inscribed in or upon the body itself.

The spread of confession fascinated Foucault (1990, 59), who saw it as having come to encompass fields as diverse as 'justice, medicine, education, family relationships, and love relations...the most ordinary affairs of everyday life'. Whether it be in the context of a therapeutic relationship, in a spiritual or forensic setting, in a romantic relationship or on television, confession involves a relation of power between the confessor and confessor. As Foucault goes on to say:

> Confession is a ritual of discourse...that unfolds within a power relationship, for one does not confess without the presence (or virtual

presence) of a partner who is not simply the interlocutor but the authority who requires the confession, prescribes and appreciates it, and intervenes in order to judge, punish, forgive, console, and reconcile; a ritual in which the…expression alone, independently of its external consequences, produces intrinsic modifications in the person who articulates it: it exonerates, redeems, and purifies him; it unburdens him of his wrongs, liberates him, and promises him salvation… Its veracity is not guaranteed by the lofty authority of the magistery, nor by the tradition it transmits, but by the bond, the basic intimacy in discourse, between the one who speaks and what he is speaking about. On the other hand, the agency of domination does not reside in the one who speaks (for it is he who is constrained), but in the one who listens…and this discourse of truth finally takes effect, not in the one who receives it, but in the one from whom it is wrested. (Foucault 1990, 61–2)

The hapless guest on a talk show, the client in the consulting room and the diligent reader of self-help literature are hailed by demands that they confess on the premise that the fundamental qualities of their condition must be somehow painfully owned up to. In confessing then, there is a kind of abasement or contrition, yet it is through confession that the self is produced. The expression of the self and the discourse of who one might be is, on the one hand, called into being through this process of subjugation, yet on the other is supposed to represent a kind of freedom. The person who has been confessed and who has subjected him or herself to that particular discipline or labour has been somehow emancipated. This can be seen in the process of psychotherapy, counselling and self-help. They subject the individual to a process of confession, all the way from painful childhood experiences in the past to dysfunctional thinking in the present, from acknowledgement of hitherto improperly recognized 'needs' to expunging feelings of shame; the confessional process will set us free. Even for those of us whose paternity has been exposed on daytime television, we are somehow better off for having this truth disclosed. The process of disclosure is part of becoming 'who we really are'.

Selves, Identities, Consumption and Brands

The verbal confession alone is only part of this perpetual self-scrutiny and chronic self-disclosure of the individual under advanced liberalism. The places we are seen, the company we keep and the merchandise with which we surround ourselves are part of the process too.

The idea of self-display as an important component of identity has been explored extensively in literature on youth and youth subcultures. The process of building identity through artefacts, fashions and styles of music may be particularly conspicuous among adolescents. Both classic and contemporary writers on this stage of life see it as involving a process whereby youths both individuate from their parents and identify themselves within social peer groups (Deutsch and Theodorou 2010; Erikson 1959, 1968; Harter 1999). Yet with decreased financial options and limitations on the likely remuneration in the labour market, constructing an identity that meets the expectations of individualistic consumer culture becomes more complex. The increased focus on consumerism as a means of building individual identity comes at a time when the gap between low- and high-income households is widening (Deutsch and Theodorou 2010). Consequently, signifiers of luxury, wealth and prestige take on a special significance. Pattillo-McCoy (1999, 146) noted in her study of Black youth in Chicago, that the youths

> use their own bodies and the accessories that adorn them as status markers and symbols of identity…[they are] walking mega-malls forever trying to stay in material dialogue with their friends as well as their enemies.

The ongoing and increasing salience of fashion brands in young people's discourse has been widely noted (Pilcher 2011), and children routinely and knowingly use their consumer awareness in self-positioning and identity construction. As Bennett (2011) remarks, the industries of culture, fashion and media celebrate, shape and are shaped by the evolution of youth identity. This itself is, in late modernity, more likely to represent intersections of taste, aesthetics and affectivity, rather than earlier bonds of social class interest or community. As Bennett (2011) and Chaney (1996) before him have argued, youth identities are part of a kind of creative project. This is akin to what Callinicos (1989) termed 'postmodern dandyism' in a 'supermarket of style'. Self-disclosure through the body, through our accessories and through our speech, identifies who we are and what our worth in the social marketplace might be.

With the proliferation of ways in which we might confess or disclose ourselves, from clothing choices, bodily idioms or hexis, our televised confessions or our therapeutic outpourings, comes an associated requirement to distinguish the quality of those confessions. Some of them are less valid or valuable than others. Some may be themselves symptoms of a continued pathology rather than revealing something authentic about the self. Self-assemblage or self-disclosure through patterns of consumption is often considered to be less valuable and, in some cases, even unhealthy by many commentators.

The idea that consumption itself is associated with malaise and even illness has been gaining ground over the past decade. The notion that enjoying consumer goods leads to so-called 'affluenza' has been proposed in a number of books, such as the eponymous *Affluenza* by Oliver James (2007), Hamilton and Denniss' *Affluenza: When Too Much is Never Enough* (2005) or *Affluenza: The All Consuming Epidemic* (de Graaf, Wann et al. 2001). For James, (2007, 43) affluenza involves 'placing a high value on money, possessions, appearances (physical and social) and fame' and this becomes the driving force of the (alleged) increasing rate of mental illness in English-speaking societies. James is fond of maintaining that English-speaking nations have twice the rate of mental disorder as those in mainland Europe. Economists Eaton and Eswaran (2009, 1088) describe the essential enigma:

> While economic growth has led to substantial increases in per capita real incomes, there have been no corresponding increases in average subjective well-being.

Within the social sciences themselves, there is considerable agreement with the basic premise of affluenza. Economic data purporting to demonstrate material increases in living standards is contrasted with information about dissatisfactions and mental ill health. There is considerable concern in so-called positive psychology about the impact of materialism and the limitations of hedonism and the blind pursuit of money (Christopher and Hickinbottom 2008). Or, as one of the founder members of the positive psychology movement asked, 'if we're so rich why aren't we happy?' (Csikszentmihalyi 1999, 821). Expressing oneself through artefacts, possessions or desiderata indicative of improved living standards then, is inferior and representative of at least crassness or perhaps even pathology. Only certain kinds of disclosures are granted therapeutic or self-enhancing benefits.

Much of this discussion, of course, presupposes that affluence itself has already been achieved. Yet when we examine the circumstances of much everyday life, we are just as likely to find that materialism and hedonism seem a distant dream. The UK's Office for National Statistics' Annual Survey of Hours and Earnings (2010) reports that of the 21,300,000 jobs included, the median gross annual pay earned was just over £21,300. If full-time jobs alone (of which there were just over 15,600,000) are considered, median gross annual pay was £25,900. To give some idea of how far from affluence this is, the BBC reported in November 2010 that average house prices in the UK were £246,387, based on Land Registry data, suggesting that typical annual wage levels were around one tenth the price of a house (BBC 2010c). These examples could be multiplied across a variety of items of income and expenditure, but two nails should suffice to attach the sign.

The profusion of material about the futility of material improvements in living standards has proceeded in the absence of detailed study of the texture of materially impoverished everyday life. Overarching national measures of economic activity are pitted against anecdotes about exemplary individuals who are wealthy but unhappy. The pursuit of purported 'affluenza' is not followed through down to measures of individual or household income. Thus, a good deal of the writing about the disadvantages of wealth provides intellectual support for the lowering of expectations and the governance of conduct away from securing material comforts and towards the idea that a sense of self should properly come through the confessional rearrangement of one's internal mental architecture.

In much of the literature about affluenza, and a good deal of scholarship on the rewards of one's career, human activity or work is described as if it were not primarily about economic or material advances for oneself or one's family, but instead is formulated as properly being about work upon the self, or an introspective fascination with the work process itself. As James (2007, 298) says 'the key is to examine what it is about your work that you find truly interesting, and put that before pay and promotion'. This echoes Csikszentmihalyi (1997), who argued that individuals find fulfilment in everyday life when they achieve a balance between their capabilities and skills, their aspirations and the challenges they face. In this formulation, self-fulfilling activities are those that engross the individual and divert consciousness away from oneself. Csikszentmihalyi called this experience 'achieving flow'. When the challenge is greater than the skills available, the result is an uncomfortable level of anxiety. Alternatively, when skill levels are high but the challenge low, then boredom is said to be likely. Thus fulfilment comes not primarily from the fruits of achieving an aspiration, but also from the process of releasing potentialities (Rantala and Lehtonen 2001). Work too then is a form of confession, a kind of self-disclosure, such that the citizen's potentialities are disclosed to him or herself. Through reflection on our work, we discover what is really important to us and thus in a fundamental sense who we are.

But this is not all. There are implications here for how we think about welfare and wellbeing. Wellbeing, rather than concerning the sovereignty of the individual regarding his or her own judgement about what is valuable, or the notion of 'agent sovereignty' as Arneson (1999) called it, is bounded and constrained. Certain kinds of labours or confessions are of greater value; some meditations on the wellsprings of the good life are worthy of nurturance and others are pathological. The most valuable confessions and self-developments in this view involve the individual in foreswearing material advantage and placing him or herself in a pupil-like relationship to expertise, an obeisance in front of those who hear our confessions, and expressing a willingness to be reconfigured through labour. These are purportedly the things that genuinely facilitate self-actualization, or the process of becoming who we really are. The sovereignty of the individual therefore goes hand in hand with the operation of larger powers and attempts to shape selves and identities in line with grander neoliberal projects. A self which is apt to defer to expertise, to seek development in inner directed transformation and confession rather than demands for increased living standards or possessions, and to see work as a therapeutic rather than an economic process, is one agreeable to many potential employers as well as to actual and prospective governments.

Whilst it may be that there are limits to the structures within which it is possible or permitted to exercise agent sovereignty, it is equally possible to detect increasingly common directions in which the self may be developed as a commodity. A striking example of the commodification of the self and the entrepreneurial project comes in the vogue for using marketing techniques as a means of self-enhancement. The entrepreneurial project of the self takes on its most assertive aspect in people who describes themselves as 'brands'. This phrase, with its allied conception of the self as a self-manufactured commercial product, seems to have been first used by American short story writer and novelist John Cheever (1912–1982) of whom it was reported that

> by the time of his death in 1982, Cheever had become 'a literary elder statesman' in America. 'I'm a brand name,' he used to say, 'like cornflakes, or shredded wheat'. (Carpenter 1991, 17)

More recently, Martha Stewart, so-called 'goddess of domestic perfection', was reported to have said:

> 'We are creating an omnimedia presence – I'm a brand,' she boasted, on signing the deal which made Martha Stewart into a division of Time Inc. (Walker 1996, 2)

The branding of the self and making oneself central to the product was to continue into the twenty-first century. Further developments of the concept were attributed to Brit Art artist Damien Hirst. This represented a particularly novel application of the concept, because as a result of his growing fame and wealth he no longer made any of his art works himself, instead employing teams of fabricators and members of his family to make them for him. Thus the analogy with commercial production was more apposite and perhaps more telling:

> 'I think becoming a brand name is a really important part of life,' says Mr Hirst. 'It's the world we live in. It's got to be addressed, understood

and worked out, as long as you don't become your own idea of yourself, you don't start making Damien Hirsts.' (Glass and Moreton 2001, 11)

The idea of oneself as a brand has now become more widespread and borders on becoming a cliché. A further example was attributed to socialite and hotel heiress Paris Hilton. Maclean (2006, 22) reported the following conversation with her:

PH: ...everything I do is successful
Maclean: Why is that?
PH: Because I make the right choices, and I'm a brand like no one else. And I have good taste.

The idea that one is a brand invites a peculiar kind of relationship with the merchandise. On the one hand, the individual is merged with the merchandise that bears their name such that the latter is infused with the former, even though, as with Hirst's sculpture or Hilton's make-up range, they have not made it themselves. Equally therefore, it denotes a separation. The artwork, the fragrance or the handbag is not the celebrity, and by saying that they are merely a brand, they are in a sense disowning or distancing themselves from the objects that bear their name. The idea of a person as a brand suggests also that the identity or personhood is saleable. Hilton herself was the subject of a £22 million lawsuit from HairTech International because, whilst contracted to wear and promote their product which bore her name, she did not do so (BBC 2010d). Thus the relationship between the person as the brand and the goods is complex and sometimes tenuous – the sutures between them are attenuated or augmented by legal action, claim and counterclaim. Nevertheless, the relationship between the self as brand and the merchandise facilitates both the promotion of self and the promotion of goods.

The sense of the self as a kind of product goes on at a variety of levels within the economy. Whilst the commercially successful and their goods can be brands, there is also the more mundane way in which the rest of us can invest ourselves with the skills, knowledge and aesthetic qualities to make us 'employable' (Baker and Brown 2007). The idea of being a brand is clearly a seductive prospect. In autumn 2010 the UK's business game show *The Apprentice* featured a young man who claimed that he was 'Stuart Baggs the brand'. His boast was not taken seriously on the programme, yet for a short time became as much of a catch phrase as host Alan Sugar's 'you're fired'. In more mundane contexts, 'workplace assessments and job interviews increasingly demand that the candidate explicitly trumpets his or her strengths' (McCartney 2010b, 28). In other words, this is indicative of a wider trend.

Fortunately, there is assistance available in the form of career self-help books. Whilst Stuart Baggs was ridiculed, he was merely acting on the advice of Tom Peters (1997) or Purkiss and Royston-Lee (2009) in their book *Brand You*. In this, they advise people on how to make an impression and leave the audience, whether this involves colleagues, superiors or prospective employers, with a distinctive message about who you are and what you can do. Yet in this self-branding there is a grounding in authenticity too. As Duits and Vis (2009) note, the value of 'authenticity' is pervasive in the evaluation of selves, celebrities and moral actors. External moral precepts are perhaps less important than the question of whether a person is being true to themselves (Dyer 1991). Thus, the personal brand has to be something you 'evoke naturally' (Purkiss and Royston-Lee 2009, 89) and the image you project should be 'authentic' (2009, 73). Self-branding and presenting yourself as a brand is about identifying and enhancing who you authentically are. As Bourdieu (1990, 12) puts it, these self-branded social agents are 'virtuosos' of practice, drawing creatively upon a 'sense' of how to behave which derives not from 'conscious, constant rules, but practical schemes'. Like many of the other practices and processes that we have described, the branding process evokes the idea that there is a genuine, authentic core within the individual that is as much dispositional as it is reflexive (Bottero 2010), that can be coaxed into being through this process of pupillage, self-help and career counselling.

Conclusion: Producing, Confessing and Branding the Self

Thinking across the various themes that we have addressed in this chapter, several features seem to be common. The first is that the self is a kind of production. A form of labour accumulates the capital of the self through a variety of forms of work. Yet in much popular culture and popular advice at least, this is not seen as a form of fabrication that may freely yield any possible form of self. The labour is about realizing what is already there in embryonic form, a drawing forth or self-actualization. With the erosion of two-tiered views of the human condition and the substitution of a single-tiered ontology, the self and in particular its authenticity disclosed through confession, becomes the touchstone of value and morality. At the same time, the idea of confession in one form or another has apparently survived intact from the traditional to the post-traditional world. Through the ubiquity of confession, in therapy, on daytime television, through our bodily hexis and pursuit of fashion, our self-branding and in connection with friendships and supportive collegial relationships, we are allegedly brought more fully into contact with our real selves.

Over and above the kind of self-disclosure elicited in these confessions of the self, it is apposite to note some of the power relationships involved. The person hearing the confession has a kind of tutelary relationship with the person making the confession, whilst the person confessing resembles a pupil or apprentice, for whom

> the relationship to the master who holds the secrets is of paramount importance; only he, working alone, can transmit this art in an esoteric manner and as the culmination of an initiation in which he guides the disciple's progress with unfailing skill and severity. The effects of this masterful art...are said to transfigure the one fortunate enough to receive its privileges: an absolute mastery of the body, a singular bliss, obliviousness to time and limits, the elixir of life, the exile of death, and its threats. (Foucault 1990, 58)

Detraditionalization has not necessarily brought freedom in a simple libertarian sense, but has instead offered a variety of forms of apprenticeship or pupillage which can be chosen by the individual as paths through which to activate and actualize tendencies that, so the logic goes, *must* have authenticity present deep inside the self already. The rituals of truth through which it is evoked, cultivated, branded and capitalized are not overtly brutal coercive practices, but rather involve an *ascetic* practice of self-formation. Here we use the term ascetic following Foucault, to mean an 'exercise of self upon the self by which one attempts to develop and transform oneself and to attain a certain mode of being' (Foucault 1997, 282). This 'work' undertaken upon the self might, in popular discourse, imply that there is a hidden self or inner nature or essence that has been 'concealed, alienated, or imprisoned in and by mechanisms of repression' (Foucault 1997, 282), that is somehow liberated through this process of work, confession and capitalization. This is work that will set one free to be who one wants to be. The self is meticulously produced in a variety of 'projects of docility' (Foucault 1977, 136). These projects are enacted in the form of institutional practices, but they are guided by the modern quest for the authentic 'truth' of the self.

The process of self-development, whilst compatible with individualism and with detraditionalized self-aware personhood, is also profoundly compatible with the vicissitudes of the market under conditions of neoliberalism. It is a self continually in thrall to expertise, to therapeutic authority and to the development of the self itself. Material shifts in the individual's circumstances are downplayed or even seen as unhealthy in favour of the notion that work should properly be a labour upon the self and involve the pursuit of fulfilment. The alignment of the individual with the vocabularies, concepts and disciplines of the market is discussed as if it were a deepening of personal authenticity, in the form of self-branding. The individual is regulated as markets are deregulated, relocalized within specific tutelary relationships as capital is globalized and self-capitalized as public services are decapitalized.

Chapter Nine

TALKING CITIZENSHIP INTO BEING

Introduction: The Fulfilled, Responsible Citizen

In this final chapter we will consider how citizenship is at present talked about and show how these current discourses fit with the kinds of issues discussed earlier in this book. We have talked of citizens throughout this volume, but in this chapter we will extend some of the reflections on citizenship with which we began at the outset, exploring some of the kinds of citizenship discussed and the relationship with which citizens are being brought into with one another and with themselves. Olson's (2008, 40) definition of citizenship as pertaining to the 'status of individuals in relation to a political unit' could embrace political units or polities in the form of regimes comprising impersonal institutions and offices involved in governance, as well as political units comprised of publics, political movements or communities. As we have seen, both strands may be activated in contemporary manifestations of responsibilization, with exhortations from policymakers on the one hand and movements of citizens themselves on the other. These citizens might, for example, be desirous of undertaking therapy, self-help or participating in health screening schemes.

As Perron et al. (2010) describe, citizenship could be conceptualized as a right or an entitlement, a responsibility, a status, a practice, a process and an outcome. In addition, it is sometimes formulated as a 'reciprocal relationship between the state and individuals' (George, Lee et al. 2003, 71). Condor (2011) reminds us that attempts to understand citizenship are characterized by disagreement and citizenship constitutes an exemplary instance of what Gallie (1956, 169) termed an 'essentially contested' concept: an idea which is complex, normatively laden, and which involves 'endless disputes about [its] proper use'.

As we have argued so far, much contemporary discussion of the relationship between the state apparatuses and the individual calls upon the citizen to be a self-sufficient and self-realizing subject, one who can master their own conduct so as to make wise choices as to the course of action to pursue and to make appropriate decisions to achieve particular goals. Such activities may be concerned with the management of one's wealth, one's conduct in social space, one's duties as an actual or potential employee or as a voter. Yet this is not to place the citizen in a position of full autonomy. For as Shotter (1993, 134–5) argues, the practices of citizenship operate within the 'contradictory, ambivalent, and indeterminate time-space of negotiation'. As we have seen in the preceding chapters, the focus on a self-reliant individual is accompanied by an apparently countervailing focus on the extent that individuals should act in accordance with a variety of advice from policymakers and experts, and know themselves not by first-hand knowledge but through submitting themselves to a variety of medical and therapeutic processes to supplement, or even supervene, over any personal guesses they might have about how they are feeling.

In much of the contemporary policy that we have discussed, a key theme concerns the way in which the personal has been linked with the collective, effectively problematizing the erstwhile popular dichotomy between the private and the public spheres: 'Self-fulfilment is no longer a personal or a private goal…[It] is something we owe to society' (Cruikshank 1999, 89). Issues that might once have been matters of private preference – what we eat, how we manage our health or how we bring up children – are now part of a welfare state enmeshed in the political toil to promote empowerment, responsibility and active citizenship (Clarke 2005; McKee and Cooper 2008).

As coalition prime minister David Cameron was reported to say at the Conservative Party Conference in 2010: 'Citizenship isn't a transaction – in which you put your taxes in and get your services out. It's a relationship – you're part of something bigger than yourself, and it matters what you think and you feel and you do' (D'Ancona 2010, 24). David Cameron has thus sought to redefine fairness not just as an egalitarian question, but one linked to a notion of behaviour and just desserts, stating: 'For too long we have measured success in tackling poverty by the size of the cheque we give people. We say: let us measure our success by the chances we give' (Wintour 2010, 1).

This 'mattering' of thoughts, feelings and conduct has accompanied a withdrawal from earlier ambitions to reduce poverty in material or monetary terms and instead substitute a polity of thoughts, feelings and 'chances'. In tandem with this there is a growing tacit consensus in 'citizenship talk' in both scholarly and lay literature that a framework focused on citizenship will bring on the achievement of patient or consumer healthcare rights (Perron, Rudge et al. 2010). The idea of health as something that we consume has become central to many strategies for intervening upon collective existence in the name of life and health as well as modes of subjectification, in which individuals work on themselves in the name of individual or collective health enhancement (Rabinow and Rose 2006).

As we have remarked, whilst all this is happening a further trend in the politics of conduct is that policymakers are increasingly relying not on any clear popular mandate, but instead on expertise to advise, educate and shape the citizen. Richard Thaler, one of the authors of the popular book on persuasion and behaviour change *Nudge* (Thaler and Sunstein 2008), is an advisor to David Cameron's Behavioural Insight Team. Deputy prime minister Nick Clegg was reported as saying 'The challenge is to find ways to encourage people to act in their own and in society's long-term interest, while respecting individual freedom' (Tyler 2011, 6). As Condor (2011) notes, appeals to citizenship on the part of policymakers typically involve some reference to psychological states and processes, such as identity, opinions, values, understanding and aspirations. It is this terrain that has become the subject of expanded interest on the part of policymakers, experts on happiness and specialists in the governance of conduct. To turn once again to Rose and Miller (2010), personal autonomy is not the opposite of political power but 'a key term of its exercise'. To us, one of the most striking features of the turn in policy in contemporary life is the preoccupation with both the micromanagement of conduct and the preoccupation with the interior world of the citizen. This contrasts with what might have been called the concern with the bodily capital – addressed through powdered milk, vitamin enhanced orange juice and inoculation programmes – that were found in the immediate postwar welfare programmes.

The interior world of the citizen, which might have previously been beyond the reach of the public sphere, perhaps previously a matter of everyday proprioceptive awareness, where problems were solved with localized ingenuities and unreflective cultural commonplaces, is now a matter of 'choice' or 'lifestyle' as well as one where expertise may be deployed. Despite the confusions and contradictions of neoliberalism which we outlined at the outset, and the difficulties of the concept when applied to contemporary economic policy, there remains a profound legacy of the movement when it comes to the psychological sphere:

> For neo-liberalism the political subject is less a social citizen with powers and obligations deriving from membership of a collective body, than an individual whose citizenship is active. This citizenship is to be manifested not in the receipt of public largesse, but in the energetic pursuit of personal fulfilment and the incessant calculations that are to enable this to be achieved. (Rose and Miller 2010, 298)

Neoliberalism then has not necessarily succeeded in paving the way towards a low taxation, 'small government', low intervention mode of governance, but the neoliberal age has been characterized by the reorganization of political rationalities so as to align them with contemporary technologies of government. These new initiatives often take the form of exhortations toward responsibility, an attempted 'autonomization' of entities from the state, and the proliferation of a multitude of calculative and managerial locales, concerned with parenting, health screening, justice, offender management, housing, community cohesion and the like. Combined with this – and a corollary of it – there is an autonomization of the state from direct control over, and responsibility for, the actions and calculations of individuals, healthcare bodies, welfare organizations, charitable bodies and other non-government organizations, as well as a degree of autonomization of these functions from the democratic mandate itself.

To citizens in advanced liberal states in the twenty-first century, these changes have been so pervasive that it is now hard to imagine how our parents' or grandparents' generation navigated the problems of life without being persuaded to conduct their lives in expert approved ways by governments, experts, health promotion agencies and a variety of devolved powers exercised by bodies concerned with matters such as school meals, supermarket sales of alcohol and healthcare issues.

From our point of view, the critical study of citizenship means examining the production of certain types of knowledges, including knowledge of the self and what counts in terms of identities, categories and relationships (Rose 1999). As Rose suggests (1999, 29–30), the task here is to 'analyse the way a word…functions in connection with other things, what it makes possible, the surfaces, networks and circuits around which it flows, the affects and passions that it mobilizes and through which it mobilizes'.

The imbrication of citizenship with persuasion, education and advice represents what Ian Hunter (1996, 149) presciently called 'the pedagogical state'. Here, one need only think of 'extended schools', 'parenting orders', ASBOs and Tony Blair's discourse of 'respect' for examples of the way in which educational principles have been extended into wider society in a process that Pykett (2007) refers to as infantilization. Associated with these notions is the idea that the citizenry is 'predictably irrational' and can be somehow nudged into prescribed courses of conduct by expert manipulation of cues that constitute their 'choice architecture' (Jones, Pykett et al. 2011). As Jones et al. comment, it is clear that this 'soft paternalism' or 'avuncular' governance is becoming more commonplace and raises important questions about democracy itself.

The actions of citizens, their everyday performances of conduct and the mindset that accompanies this are crucial to the idea of good citizenship (Pykett, Jones et al. 2010), such that acts of citizenship become normative and normalizing. As Hardin (2001, 16) notes:

Rewards…are measured out for behaviours considered socially permissible. Paradoxically, one of those rewards is being considered normal. To avoid the consequences of being labelled abnormal, and to secure rewards in our culture, people learn to monitor their interactions within a prescribed set of normative standards.

Being normal is, in an important sense, about appearing to be the captain of one's own ship. Freedom and the struggle against constraints and the desire to constantly reconfigure oneself, one's circumstances and one's livelihood are part of an insistent individualized identity project. The framing and assemblage of these virtues, habits and competencies, and how they are attributed to the responsible individual is, as White (2005, 474) says, vital to 'how the character of the good citizen is governed'.

As many other authors have noted, science, knowledge and expertise are determining features of the process by which individuals become – or are 'made' – citizens, that is, formations of knowledge are the means by which citizens are 'produced' (Cruikshank 1999; Foucault 2002; Perron, Rudge et al. 2010; Rose 2007).

> Freedom in the regime of liberalism is not a given, it is not a ready-made region which has to be respected. Freedom is something that is constantly produced. Liberalism is not an acceptance of freedom; it proposes to manufacture it constantly, to arouse and produce it, with of course [the] constraints and the problems of cost raised by this production. (Foucault 2008, 65)

Following Foucault, we would argue that the techniques with which we examine and operate upon social phenomena helps to constitute those very phenomena themselves. The practices of liberal government revolve around the categorization and management of individuals, of whom only a small minority are governed as if they are indeed capable of exercising appropriate freedoms (Dean 2007, 118–22; Pykett, Jones et al. 2011).

The neoliberal citizen, self-reliant, constantly self-reinventing and perpetually enterprising is an austere being. Even his or her enjoyment is measured against the objectives of fulfilment, fitness or perhaps the achievement of an elusive 'work-life balance'. In the next subsection, we will illustrate the reach of these new ways of thinking of citizenship by extending Novas and Rose's (2000) notion of the 'somatic citizen' to consider how we think of ourselves as biological beings and biopolitical citizens. This management of our bodies and the accompanying imperative to see ourselves as biological systems in need of scrutiny, expert advice and self-help has become ever more pervasive as a result of the processes of responsibilization (Roberts 2006).

The Rule of Expertise: Thinking of Ourselves as Biopolitical Citizens

Thinking of ourselves as responsible for our trajectory as responsible somatic citizens is not necessarily passed down in a straightforward fashion from policymaker to citizen. Under initiatives from the coalition government, the authority to shape forms of being, modes of consciousness and conduct is devolved to a variety of other sites, away from the government itself. Employers are being asked to play a part in the government's efforts to 'nudge' citizens towards more healthy lifestyles. The Department of Health wants companies to formally promote public health messages around alcohol consumption, drug use, fitness levels and eating habits (Tyler 2011, 6). Messages concerning the appropriate attitude, demeanour and course of conduct to pursue as a biosomatic citizen are found in a whole variety of places.

To illustrate the role of imperatives towards self-management, let us consider the role of pharmacological interventions in mental health, where these kinds of pressures and exhortations can be seen in action. The website of Zyprexa, an antipsychotic drug manufactured by Eli Lilly (2009), provides an apt example. It describes schizophrenia in the following way to family and friends of persons who are diagnosed:

> From the start, it's critical for you to recognize that your family member or friend's mental illness is not your fault, nor is it their fault. They are suffering from a very real – and treatable – illness that is rooted in the chemistry of their brain.

Formulating mental health problems in neurochemical terms originated not with biomedical research itself but with pharmaceutical companies. The assertions of non-culpability and inevitability accompanying this kind of account of the problem segue neatly to another kind of responsibility for the patient and their carers, that of the responsibility of managing one's mental disorder, that does indeed frequently fall to the patient and their family members (Rose 2007). This includes complying with treatment as directed by an expert such as a healthcare practitioner. The duty then is to make oneself (or one's relative) a functioning or at least socially acceptable member of society.

Seeing ourselves in terms of neurones may be becoming a duty of biomedical citizenship, since failure to think about our brains in neuroscientific terms – or at all – not only invites risk but may increasingly constitute moral failure (Pitts-Taylor 2010, 649). Biological vitality, from the levels of surface flesh all the way to molecule, neurone and gene, has become a prime resource for 'marketization' in biocapitalist economies (Waldby and Cooper 2008, 58).

In a paper by Simone Fullagar (2009), women who take anti-depressant medications were seen as having *allowed* themselves to be neurologically deficient. The power relations of depression diagnosis demand neurochemical treatment; without it, women are seen as lacking in self-care: 'The neurochemically deficient self is…required to exercise responsibility and self-control to restore and maximize their life potential via biomedical expertise' (Fullagar 2009, 403).

As Rose elaborates:

I suggest that a neurochemical sense of ourselves is increasingly being layered onto other, older senses of the self, and invoked in particular settings and encounters with significant consequences… To grasp the world in this way is to imagine the disorder as residing within the individual brain and its processes, and to see psychiatric drugs as a first line intervention, not merely for symptom relief but for ways of modulating and managing these neurochemical anomalies. (Rose 2007, 222–3)

The 'chemical imbalance' theory of mental disorders is hard to sustain from a fine grained reading of available research (Dean 2011; France, Lysaker et al. 2007) and some medications may instead be addressing social disadvantage rather than a discrete disorder per se (Isaacs 2006). It is not our purpose to undertake a thorough critique here or suggest that scepticism is necessarily more truthful than acceptance of this view. Rather, what is at stake here is the tendency to see the tasks of citizenship or patienthood (which often amounts to the same thing) in terms of a task of managing oneself as a corporeal entity. The neurochemical self is just one example, of course. We could just as easily explore the hormonal citizen and the implied necessity of managing oneself as a hormonal entity (Roberts 2006). These examples resonate with the others that we have given earlier in this volume about the healthcare matrix in which a new diagram is emerging of the relationships between the susceptibility, risk, preemption, precaution and self-management of a variety of potential hazards of being human. From the management of neurochemistry and hormones, through to the gross anatomical features such as body size and shape and dietary stipulations which are still at large, the territory of management has extended inwards to the imagined neuronal or molecular level.

This expanded reach of health and responsibility for one's wellbeing at a biological level has extended into many other activities which might not primarily have been thought of as medical interventions at all. For example, for many decades in Wales people have enjoyed singing in choirs and competitively in festivals such as *eisteddfodau*, as well as in religious worship. Even opera in Wales is a somewhat less elitist pursuit than in England and

Welsh opera singers such as Bryn Terfel still reside in the area in which they grew up. However, the *Western Mail* recently featured an article informing readers that singing helps decrease stress. Also, 'for people with dementia and those who care for them it is particularly rewarding. It's amazing how when other memories start to fade, songs loved from younger days remain' (*Western Mail* 2010, 24). An enthusiastic proponent is quoted as claiming 'Singing for the brain is brilliant'. Even in Wales – the proverbial 'land of song' – singing is now reconstructed and promoted as an activity that is healthful and neurologically restorative. As far as this story goes, the healthful citizen has eclipsed the citizen who is interested in music for aesthetic reasons or for enjoyment – the activity of singing is engaged in for its health giving properties. Of course this goes hand in hand with a whole range of more scientifically formulated knowledge claims about the salutogenic effects of music (Batt-Rawden and Tellnes 2011) and its abilities to bring communities together (Washington and Beecher 2011). This recasting of recreation and aesthetics in terms of health can be seen across a range of activities that might once have been viewed more exclusively in terms of having enjoyable or aesthetic qualities. Activities such as sport (Collins 2010) are now reconceptualized and compete for their share of a dwindling public purse on the basis that they promote health, raise awareness or enhance social inclusion.

The effects of this kind of practice extend into the consciousness of the individual citizen. What might once have been unreflective enjoyment is now part of the portfolio of activity for the responsible citizen, who must engage in a constant monitoring of health, a constant work of modulation, adjustment and improvement in response to the changing requirements of the practices of his or her mode of everyday life (Rose 2007, 223). All this is accomplished in and through a variety of agencies. As Rose (1993, 285) states, political rule would not itself set out the norms of individual conduct but would install and empower a variety of 'professionals' who would do so instead, investing them with authority to act as experts in the devices of social rule.

Responsibilizing the Citizen and Deresponsibilizing Public Agencies

As citizens themselves are increasingly responsibilized there is a corresponding retraction on the part of the agencies that once might have been seen as providing a service to safeguard the health and welfare of the individual (Pykett, Jones et al. 2011). New ways of conceptualizing the citizen are perhaps best understood in terms of how they are put to work (Vrecko 2010). There are a variety of ways in which the degrees of responsibility of professionals and agencies involved are contested.

One source of evidence as to how these divestments of responsibility play out in practice is the debates that occur along with the claims and counter-claims that are made in cases where a tragedy has happened. This has become increasingly evident in inquiry reports, tribunal rulings, press releases and comments made by statutory agencies in the wake of recent scandals and tragedies of the kind in which some responsibility might be attributed to healthcare or safeguarding services. For example, in May 2005, 13-month-old Aaron Gilbert was beaten to death by his mother's boyfriend Andrew Lloyd, who was subsequently imprisoned for murder. Aaron's mother was imprisoned for 'familial homicide for failing to protect her son' (BBC 2006). The authority involved, Swansea Social Services, was subject to extensive criticism both in relation to Aaron Gilbert's death and a number of other tragedies and the authority was deemed to be so troubled that the Welsh Assembly government intervened (N. Williams 2009). In relation to Aaron Gilbert, one social worker was dismissed by Swansea Council and subsequently struck off after admitting misconduct, the circumstances being that the social services team had received two anonymous phone calls expressing concern about Aaron's family days before his killing, yet the social worker had failed to respond. She was deemed to have put the baby 'at risk' and had shown 'extremely poor judgement'. Thus, the first phase of this involved an attribution of responsibility to the front line social worker. This may invite a variety of questions about the relative culpability of the person in question, the organization and the managers within it, but the service responsibility seems to have been established. Yet, as events transpired there was subsequently a mitigated deflection of responsibility back to the mother and her partner.

The social worker appealed against the decision to sack her and strike her off and won. In its ruling, the Care Standards Tribunal that reinstated her included the following comments:

> ...a number of child deaths have generated expensive enquiries looking at how agencies can do better to protect children from murder by their parents and carers. Through cases such as Kimberley Carlisle and Tyra Henry through the Victoria Climbie case to Baby Peter society has tried to understand how the deaths occurred to prevent future deaths. Alongside this has grown a culture of blame not toward those who perpetrate the crimes but toward the professionals doing their best to protect children. Yet despite the increased levels of hysteria homicide rates have remained relatively consistent over the years. People will continue to kill children despite, not because of, the efforts of professionals. No system can prevent desperate, inadequate or depraved people abusing their children. (Tribunals Service 2009, 12–13)

After this ruling, a spokesman for Swansea Council issued a statement which included the following:

> As the Care Standards Appeal Tribunal has said, the only people responsible for Aaron's death are Andrew Lloyd and Aaron's mother, Rebecca Lewis. It is now more than four years since the tragic death of Aaron Gilbert. Since that time policies, practices and procedures within Child and Family Services have changed immensely. Swansea Council has learned lessons and continues to learn. (BBC 2009)

This case illustrates a number of themes in the definition and attribution of responsibilities. There are a variety of agencies involved which may not, on the face of it, appear to be in accord. There is no single policy or set of decision makers who implement a decisive retraction and redefinition of responsibilities. Whilst there was agreement that the social services department and the social worker involved could have responded more speedily and effectively, the outcome of the case also serves to underscore some of the mechanisms that facilitate the process by which official bodies, tribunals and ultimately governments themselves are able to absolve themselves of the responsibilities involved and instead underscore the responsibility of the clients or 'service users'. Debate within the serious case review revolved around issues such as whether a letter had been sent to Aaron Gilbert's mother within the stipulated target number of working days after the call had been received. The emphasis was on policy and whether it was followed to the letter. In this case and many others like it, the question of how it came about that vulnerable young adults with mental health problems and troubled histories with authority and institutions had found themselves in the role of parent and step-parent with little effective support went unasked and unanswered in any of the published documentation surrounding the case. The restriction of the purview of inquiries and tribunals and the preoccupation with the detail of procedure is part and parcel of the 'social sorting' that is undertaken by many statutory agencies, such that citizens are assigned a position in the morally contoured human topography (Aas 2011).

The mechanisms of responsibility and accountability as they apply to official bodies and services are somewhat elastic and susceptible to redefinition. This has not passed without contest, of course. A case in point here is the response to the death of Baby P (later named as Peter Connelly) in August 2007 by officials in the London borough of Haringey. Although as a result of this case the director of children's services in Haringey Sharon Shoesmith was dismissed on the instructions of the then children's secretary, MP Ed Balls, the response from within the public services themselves was largely supportive of her and her team. The BBC reported that 60 head teachers in Haringey had signed a letter in support of her as the Baby P case was being reported in the press in November 2008 (BBC 2008) and Shoesmith received a 'Thinking of you' card from fellow directors of social services (Chandiramani 2010). In interviews Shoesmith has been keen to draw attention to the fact that prior to the Peter Connelly case, her department was rated positively by Ofsted reviews and that her chairing of the serious case review of Connelly's death was standard practice in the field and did not represent a conflict of interest as was claimed (Edernariam 2009). Moreover, Shoesmith claimed that the failure to identify the severity of the risk to Baby P and the extent of his injuries prior to his death was as a result of deception by his mother. She emphasized her own trauma as a result of negative publicity, hardship as a result of losing her job (Chandiramani 2010) and that her dismissal represented 'breathtaking recklessness' on the part of Ed Balls, whose decision, she said, had placed more children in danger (Moore 2009).

The response of Sharon Shoesmith, at least as it has been reported in the national and professional press, is instructive. The reliance on prior Ofsted reports as indicative of quality, the presentation of self as victim and sufferer of trauma and the positioning of oneself as a beleaguered bulwark against even worse eventualities are features of public service discourse which accompany the retreat from responsibility in the public sphere. The idea of public service managers as somehow frail or traumatized in the light of demands placed on them is increasingly discovered by students of New Public Management (Goldfinch and Wallis 2010; Walker, Brewer et al. 2011) and is a discourse deployed particularly in the face of demands for accountability. The reliance on ratings from processes of audit, inspection and review from one public service agency examining another, or from processes of self-examination and self-report is a feature not only of public service management as a whole (Walker, Brewer et al. 2011), but of healthcare work in particular (Brown and Crawford 2009; Crawford and Brown 2008). It resonates with the comments made above concerning how quality, compliance and accountability have been imbricated with procedural adherence rather than broader challenges about capability and purpose. The inconsistency inherent in judgements of organizations evaluating one another in the public service culture of audit, inspection and review is highlighted in the reported comments of Ofsted's then chief Christine Gilbert, who was quoted as suggesting that the sudden change in its opinion of Haringey's Children's Services from good to seriously inadequate was as a result of deception on the part of Haringey on earlier Ofsted visits (Curtis 2008).

Thus, even where one public body has failed to identify problems in another, the retreat from any formal grasp of responsibility is a discourse which is ready to hand as both a means of exoneration and an explanation. As we have noted above, the retreat of public bodies from responsibility is often accompanied by a reassertion of the culpability of the people who have committed the crime, consolidating the function of service bodies to undertake what Aas (2011) termed the 'sorting' process, i.e., the placing of clients or citizens in moral categories. Shoesmith was quoted as saying: 'none of the agencies involved with the family are responsible for the death. Those responsible for this tragedy have been prosecuted' (Edernariam 2009, 4). Increasingly, the response is to comment on the abdication of responsibility on the part of the client or service user, accompanied by assertions of the stress and trauma that the service itself has suffered as a result of the bad publicity. Other scholars have noted cognate processes at work in public service delivery, such that the public is often seen as comprising two different constituencies – a nice public who may be consulted and appeased and a nasty public who must be reminded of their culpability and the punishments that they are likely to incur (Clarke 2010). The apparent failures of the public services then are repackaged as this failure of the latter public, the ones who persist in irresponsible courses of action and who wilfully ignore the possibility of punishment.

The debates over responsibility in the public services, whether or not people find themselves in trouble for substandard performance, take place in an atmosphere of increased transparency and enhanced scrutiny. Ferlie, Ashburner et al. (1996) argue that the new varieties of public management have brought professionals involved in the delivery of public services under increased scrutiny and has attempted to make professional practice more transparent and controllable. Private sector notions of market forces, assessment and management have underpinned the rise of managerialism (Loewenthal 2002), audit culture (Power 1997) and 'neo-bureaucracy' (Harrison and Smith 2003) in public sector services, where economic rationalism and technicism, efficiency, accountability and performativity are privileged over basic trust in public sector professionals (O'Neill 2002). McGivern, Fischer et al. (2009) have also remarked on an 'emerging assemblage' of regulatory procedures in the field of psychotherapy and counselling. The question of responsibility is therefore less a matter of whether the official concerned has done the right thing in any moral sense, but rather whether there are policies and procedures and whether they have been followed. The transparency and media scrutiny also allow a variety of new storylines to proliferate concerning the diffusion or deflection of responsibility itself and about the personal trauma suffered by officials, practitioners and their relatives. The emphasis on scrutiny and accountability in public services has not necessarily yielded more or better services in any simple sense, but instead has made visible new territories of public management, service delivery and even the private spaces of public sector workers. Yet the focus on these interior organizational and personal spaces has proceeded in tandem with a retraction in the ambit of services themselves in important respects, away from the client groups who are seen as difficult, demanding or irresponsible. These then are the citizens who are seen as in greatest need of taking responsibility themselves.

Vulnerabilities and Failures of Responsibility

As we have argued in this volume, in tandem with the development of new arenas in which individuals are exhorted to grasp their new responsibilities, there are parallel processes going on that enhance the sense of vulnerability and fragility, where issues such as health, psychological integrity or one's skills and capabilities are concerned. Hirschorn (1997) suggests that in the face of new organizational structures, a sense of 'market risk' has emerged, creating a sense of vulnerability in individuals who 'question their own competence and their ability to act autonomously. In consequence, just when they need to build a more sophisticated psychological culture, they inadvertently create a more primitive one' (Hirschorn 1997, 27).

The diligence and meticulous self-monitoring required of the citizen under neoliberalism is not deemed to be achievable by everyone. The growing stringency applied to the individual means that an ever greater proportion of the population will fail to measure up. More people are falling into the categories which are seen to be in need of surveillance (Aas 2011) or the threat of punishment (Clarke 2010). Despite the policy emphasis on combating social exclusion and creating Big Societies, the very foundations of policy itself create the points of failure where people will fall through the net of citizenship.

An example of the trend towards the attribution of heightened vulnerability comes from Platform 51, formerly the Young Women's Christian Association, who published a report claiming that 'our research shows that in England and Wales 63% of girls and women have been affected by mental health problems of some kind' (Platform 51 2011, 2). This high figure was obtained in a poll of just over 2000 women and girls over the age of 12 and a somewhat elastic definition of mental health problems was adopted, including 'feeling sad and tearful', suffering 'low self-esteem' and 'feeling worthless' (Platform 51 2011, 5). In Wales, Platform 51 was concerned with the situation of Welsh women and demanded 'effective intervention' from the Welsh Assembly government. Platform 51 were also concerned that 'women were not identifying the issues as mental health problems' and said that 'more needed to be done to encourage self-referral' (BBC 2011a).

This expansive definition of mental health problems as well as the notion that the respondents in the survey were not sufficiently likely to identify

problems as mental health ones, goes hand in hand with an anxiety throughout
the report about young women's eating (4) and drinking (8), debt (8) and their
engagement in sexual relationships and recreational drug taking (9). The
report thus takes its place in a tradition of concern over young women on the
part of government, educators and moralists who have regularly expressed
unease over young women's 'excess' where drink, drugs, sex and consumerism
are concerned. The manoeuvre of Platform 51, now that it has transformed
itself away from its formerly religious identity, is to understand these issues as
matters of mental health rather than as primarily spiritual or moral issues.
Certainly there is an implied moral imperative on the part of the medical
profession and government agencies to act, but the individuals with whom
the report is concerned are now infused with vulnerability and fragility and
are positioned as acting through the influence of mental ill health rather than
making autonomous choices. They are, in this discourse, too vulnerable or
too damaged to be seen as exercising autonomy among the various options
and activities available to them. Thus, as well as the more academically based
studies of the epidemiology of mental health with which we began chapter
five, it is important to note that the territory of research is being colonized
by other groups and bodies keen to press their case. The notion of pervasive
vulnerability thus engendered finds its way into other initiatives and practices
which cast themselves as useful in that they can address the problems identified
in this way.

Among the variety of initiatives being pressed forward to address this
alleged vulnerability and damage we might cite the spring 2011 prospectus
produced by Bangor University's Lifelong Learning Unit, which advertises a
number of 'continuing professional development' modules suitable for 'anyone
working in the substance misuse sector or whose role…would benefit from
education and training around these subject areas'. The 'core worker skills'
module 'will increase your awareness and understanding of personal, group
and community attitudes, feelings, ideas and values and…how they affect
behavior and practice. You will develop active listening skills which enable the
building of trusting relationships, as well as developing practice which fosters
equal relationships'. The 'introduction to suicide and self-harm' module
involves discussing 'a range of biopsychosocial and therapeutic approaches'
concerned with suicide and self-harm understanding and management.
Modules are described as 'highly experiential' and participants are encouraged
to participate in 'role play'.

The description of all these modules is relentlessly upon the emotional and
behavioural world of the individual as both provider of service and recipient
of the service, with a view to reshaping that individual. 'Equal relationships'
are mentioned only in context of practice with clients. There is a striking

absence of sociopolitical perspectives, yet these modules are being taught in a region with a high suicide rate, poor services for clients with mental health and addiction problems, generations of socioeconomic disadvantage and a unique ethno-linguistic geography and heritage. This course takes its place among many other initiatives to professionalize and manage vulnerability through psychosocial means. People are prepared for careers in public service such that their focus and capabilities will be organized to address the vulnerabilities that their training has taught them to see. Whether flesh and blood clients do indeed display vulnerabilities like this is more debatable, but what is interesting here is how the likely client is formulated in training programmes for the practitioner.

Capitalizing on Vulnerability

This interplay of responsibility and vulnerability can be seen in another theme to which we have returned several times throughout this volume, namely the way that suffering can be turned into a kind of capital. So deep runs the entrepreneurialism at the heart of the subject-citizen that tragedies and hardships can be repackaged as assets to add personal credentials and to even yield monetary rewards for the individual.

There is now a whole sector of voluntary or paid employment in which part of the person specification for such posts is to have experience of a situation involving suffering in some way. Such rationale usually is based on the notion that one has to have experienced certain events to fully understand their impact or to be effective at advising others how to deal with such impact. We are thinking here of, for example, positions advertised for 'mental health advocates', 'service user representatives' or 'health trainers'. Adverts for such positions usually stipulate that one must have experienced the condition in question to be eligible to apply. Yet reading the literature produced by people employed in such positions (or even conversing with them) it is clear that credibility is not so much achieved by experiencing the condition, but by the very suffering itself that is involved. In the case of the mental health service users' movement, although the multiple deprivations and deeply distressing experiences to which most people with a serious mental health problem are subjected are now well-documented, the announcement of many new appointments continues to be accompanied by a biography in which suffering is highlighted.

One of the authors of this book was recently asked by a service users' organization if they would write their life narrative for display on this organization's website because students with mental health problems needed 'role models' of academics who had been or were 'service users'. They were not asked for their academic biography or even to dispense practical advice – the focus was to be entirely upon 'sharing' the 'terrible things' that they 'had gone through'.

The value placed on suffering as a source of stories that can be circulated and as a means of accumulating personal capital is something that we discussed earlier. However, in addition to the dispossessed and celebrities, people who have distinguished themselves in other walks of life are now contributing to the genre. One of the most fascinating recent examples of the misery memoir is that by Constance Briscoe (2006), a lawyer and judge who wrote and publicised *Ugly*, a story alleged to be closely based on her own childhood, that included the central character's mother constantly berating her for her alleged ugliness, calling her Miss Pissabed, as well as subjecting her to other serious prolonged physical and mental abuse. *Ugly* was followed by *Beyond Ugly*, marketed explicitly as the story of Constance Briscoe's later adolescence and early adulthood, describing how she underwent a substantial amount of cosmetic surgery to correct her perceived ugliness. Her story was subsequently featured in *Take a Break*, a magazine whose target audience is probably not members of the judiciary. She gave media interviews in which she described how she was still very unhappy with aspects of her appearance, particularly her feet and how she planned to undergo further cosmetic surgery to remove bones from her feet to make them smaller. At one point, Constance Briscoe became embroiled in a court battle with her mother and sister when they denounced her story as untrue. Ms Briscoe won the case among considerable media interest.

Ugly is unremarkable among the scores of misery memoirs detailing severe and degrading abuse that people suffered as children, yet what makes it so fascinating is the nature of the career that its author had embarked upon by the time she wrote it. Unique to the present era is the way that people in prominent roles in public life are increasingly likely to contribute to the genre. John Prescott, former deputy prime minister under New Labour describes his eating disorder and problems with alcohol in his co-written autobiography (Prescott and Davies 2008). Alastair Campbell (2011) former New Labour director of communications (1997–2003) describes a 'nervous breakdown', depression and alcohol problems in his published diaries.

Writing and publicising misery memoirs such as these might not have been considered appropriate or decorous in the past, yet they are now an increasingly common means of communicating about oneself or public issues (6, Radstone et al. 2006). Hence the disclosures of personal distress, misery or mental health problems on the part of those in public life, the tears on camera and the emotional interview, are part of the stock in trade of the public figure attuned to the needs of the present day communications agenda. Emotions in certain circumstances are both capitalized and capitalizing. Whilst the ordinary populace is urged to make key decisions concerning their own and their families' lives on earnestly rational grounds, on the basis of training and expert advice, the space occupied by the new emotivism in what used to be called the public sphere is expanding. Emotion is a public good which can be displayed, communicated and managed through a variety of media. Its formulation and amelioration through expertise – therapy, 'rehab', anger management, stress relief and so on – is also a part of the repertoire of good conduct demanded from the responsible citizen.

New Citizens, New Training

The outpourings of vulnerability and the outcomes of the sorting processes that disclose how many citizens are unsuited to the new climate of responsibility opens up new opportunities for investigation, training and reform. The task of rendering citizens responsible, independent and employable has itself given rise to a variety of new forms of social and economic activity. The fact that the new era of responsibility is not embraced wholeheartedly by everyone means that many public and private bodies face the task of remediating the human failure occasioned by the new challenges of citizenship. Rizq (2011) identifies these as 'social defence systems' and argues that social programmes such as the UK's policy to improve access to psychological therapies are often 'explicitly identified and tasked with what might be termed 'well-being work' and are 'underpinned by organizational structures that defend against and minimize notions of vulnerability and dependence' (Rizq 2011, 38). Having assumed a vulnerable identity, the task is then to minister to and manage that identity, either through one's own exertions or via a variety of professionalized services aimed at minimizing dependency. Once the nature of the responsible citizen is specified it becomes possible to specify also the ways in which the actual citizenry fall short, or in Clarke's (2010) terms, how official bodies seek the reform of the public as well as the reform of public services.

Hence, policymakers are concerned to start early to foster the kind of citizen that they are keen to be in governance over. In January 2011 in a UK government–commissioned report, MP Graham Allen called for a national parenting programme and regular assessments of all preschool children focusing on their 'social and emotional development', enabling 'early intervention' where necessary to 'improve the lives of vulnerable children':

There are large social benefits to intervening early, for example in terms of improvements in behaviour, reduction in violent crime, higher educational attainment, better employment opportunities and more responsible parenting of the next generation. (Allen 2011, 31)

Allen was reported as saying that 'socially and emotionally capable people are more productive, better educated, tax-paying citizens helping our nation to compete in the global economy and make fewer demands on public expenditure' (Sellgren 2011).

As we have sought to show over the course of this book, the individual under advanced liberalism cannot be allowed entirely free rein, but is subject to interventions, is trained and re-trained, 'supported', evaluated and subject to punitive sanctions including on the spot fines and a range of civil, criminal and workplace penalties and inducements if his or her behaviour departs from the prescribed ideals.

The further and higher education system is already charged with ensuring that recalcitrant individuals are re-engineered as active, 'employable' participants (Baker and Brown 2007), whereas therapies are often configured not so that greater happiness and fulfilment are possible but so that the individual can participate as a worker in the casualized, deregulated, service sector economy. Individuals are transformed into properly entrepreneurial citizens who will through judicious choices, act to maximize their 'vital capital' (their health) and the capital of the social body (Harvey 2010, 365).

As we have seen also, there is a growing industry devoted to training the carers, frontline workers, practitioners and professionals who will be working with the vulnerable, challenging and otherwise disenfranchized individuals who have fallen short of the ideals of responsible citizenship. As well as a proliferation of courses within the academy and which lead to formal qualifications, a large amount of training is delivered by émigrés from the health and social care sector who have left that line of work to deliver training and consultancy. Clarke highlights how these subjects constituted through discourses, apparatuses and practices 'do not necessarily materialize in the anticipated form' (Clarke 2005, 456). In a sense, responsibility and responsibilization facilitate a great many new roles, job descriptions and training requirements for those whose task it is to urge responsibility on others, yet they do not necessarily represent a fundamental shift in individuals' capabilities, as service users or service providers.

Technologies of Citizenship

This formation of education and training, self and mutual scrutiny is reminiscent of what Cruikshank (1999, 1) calls 'technologies of citizenship: discourses, programs and other tactics aimed at making individuals politically active and capable of self-government'. This assemblage of technologies is seen by Cruikshank as part of a more general 'will to empower'. Rather than making people powerful, the discourse of empowerment, says Cruikshank, is indicative of a concern about individuals who apparently fail to act in their own best interests and thus fall short of the fundamental properties of citizens:

> When we hear that subjects are apathetic or powerless and that citizenship is the cure, we are hearing the echo of the will to empower...I have argued that the will to empower is a strategy of government, one that seeks solutions to political problems in the governmentalization of the everyday lives of citizen subjects. (Cruikshank 1999, 122–3)

The process of responsibilization, training, support and discipline, the knowledge of the self, produced through self-scrutiny and self-monitoring techniques, can be thought of as a part of the historically localized forms of knowledge or *savoirs* discussed by Foucault (1991) that are central to his notion of governmentality. As Perron, Rudge et al. (2010) indicate, whether it is through the careful and responsible management of one's medication, joining a programme to improvement one's self-esteem, parenting skills, coping mechanisms or enhance one's anger management, the important feature is that the self is situated as an intricate part of the political, whilst at the same time being constituted as the core of the autonomous and empowered citizen. The responsibilized self becomes a responsible citizen through the application of policy, the deployment of techniques of persuasion, the help of science and government technologies that include expert intervention and thus the responsible self is brought into being (Perron, Fluet et al. 2005; Perron, Rudge et al. 2010).

Neoliberalism therefore is only partly about the design of economic life, but in important ways it is also about the design of individuals and their wellbeing. The debate about citizenship shifts the focus of concern away from macro-level questions about how we manage prosperity, vouchsafe rights, adjudicate between competing interests or raise living standards. Instead, interventions are designed and implemented in such a way as to address the individual and his or her psychic architecture. In this way, health, wellbeing and social care are nowadays about far more than the mere allocation or management of fiscal or physical resources and imply instead a form of moral assistance (Villadsen 2008) that enjoins the citizen towards full participation.

Under these circumstances, the idea of citizenship implies that the individual should have a will, a capacity for making conscious decisions and a willingness to participate in one's own and the state's affairs, in line with the stipulations of experts and policymakers. Cruikshank (1999, 1) describes how this process of asserting governance through assisting a sense of autonomy and freedom is a kind of 'technology of citizenship'. The procedures, policies, means of apportioning blame through public tribunals, rules, practices and discourses of self-responsibility and self-management allows individuals to achieve involvement and active participation in society:

> Individual subjects are transformed into citizens by what I call technologies of citizenship: discourses, programs, and other tactics aimed at making individuals politically active and capable of self-government. (Cruikshank 1999, 1)

As Perron, Rudge et al. (2010) remind us, the boundaries and practices of citizenship are fluid. Moreover they are contradictory. On the one hand, responsibility is about independence and being the captain of one's own ship. On the other it is about subsuming one's private desires and pleasures to the advice of experts. On the one hand, it is self-contained and public displays of anger and exuberance are tantamount to anti-social behaviour. On the other it is permissible – even mandatory – to emote freely in public life and to make capital and credentials out of exorbitant displays of suffering and grief. On the one hand the sufferer, service user or even the mildly unhappy citizen should avail themselves of services and expertise, but on the other we should not place too great a burden on public finances. There is increased audit, scrutiny and transparency in public services, but at the same time a withdrawal from accountability and corporate or collective responsibility. Running through all these strands is the notion of the self as an entrepreneur, constantly availing oneself of opportunities to increase one's personal capital. Equally there is an important strand of reconfiguration, reshaping and re-inscription such that it is the function of government and public service no longer to serve the needs of the people but to redesign them – the better publics described by Clarke (2010). The emergence of contemporary discourses of responsibility represents a new phase in history – the history of citizenship, of society and of the way in which we are governed.

REFERENCES

6, P., S. Radstone, C. Squire and A. Treacher. 2006. *Public Emotions*. London: Palgrave Macmillan.

Aas, K. F. 2011. '"Crimmigrant" bodies and bona fide travelers: Surveillance, citizenship and global governance'. *Theoretical Criminology* 15 (3): 331–46.

Abraham, J. 2010. 'Pharmaceuticalization of Society in Context: Theoretical, Empirical and Health Dimensions'. *Sociology* 44 (4): 603–22.

Adshead, G. 2008. 'Personal Responsibility, Abnormality, and Ethics: Psychotherapy as Moral Understanding'. *Psychiatry* 7 (5): 225–7.

All-Party Parliamentary Group on Prison Health. 2006. 'The Mental Health Problem in UK HM Prisons'. London: House of Commons.

Allen, G. 2011. *Early Intervention: The Next Steps: An Independent Report to Her Majesty's Government*. London: Cabinet Office.

Anderson, J. and A. Honneth. 2005. 'Autonomy, Vulnerability, Recognition and Justice'. *Autonomy and the Challenges to Liberalism: New Essays*, ed. J. Christman and J. Anderson, 127–49. Cambridge: Cambridge University Press.

Andrews, R. and A. Mycock. 2007. 'Citizenship Education in the UK: Divergence within a Multi-National State'. *Citizenship Teaching and Learning* 3 (1): 73–88.

Ang, I. 1985. *Watching Dallas: Soap Opera and the Melodramatic Imagination*. London: Methuen.

Angell, M. 2004. *The Truth About the Drug Companies: How They Deceive Us and What to Do About It*. New York: Random House.

Annals of Internal Medicine. 2010. http://www.annals.org/content/151/10/716.full/reply (accessed 15 April 2011).

Ap Gruffudd, G. S. 2007. 'A Study of Welsh Medium Education and Training within the National Offender Management Service in North Wales'. MA thesis, University of Wales, Bangor.

Appleby, L. 2000. 'A New Mental Health Service: High Quality and User-Led'. *British Journal of Psychiatry* 177: 290–1.

———. 2004. 'The National Service Framework for Mental Health – Five Years On'. London: Department of Health.

———. 2007. 'Mental Health Ten Years On: Progress on Mental Health Care Reform'. London: Department of Health.

Appleby, L., P. May, C. Meiklejohn, K. Edgar and I. Cummins. 2010. 'Prison Mental Health: Vision and Reality'. London: Royal College of Nursing.

Arieli, Y. 1964. *Individualism and Nationalism in American Ideology*. Cambridge, MA: Harvard University Press.

Arneson, R. J. 1999. 'Human Flourishing Versus Desire Satisfaction'. *Social Philosophy and Policy* 16 (1): 113–42.

Atkinson, W. W. 1906. *Thought Vibration: Or the Law of Attraction in the Thought World*. Chicago: The New Thought Publishing Company.

Attwood, R. 2010. 'The Principles of Confusionism'. *Times Higher Education*, 12 August.

Audit Scotland. 2009. 'Overview of Mental Health Services'. Edinburgh: Audit Scotland.

Baart, I. M. L. A. 2010. 'The Contingency of Psychiatric Genomics in a Dutch Research Consortium'. *BioSocieties* 5: 256–77.

Bacon, N., M. Brophy, N. Mguni, G. Mulgan and A. Shandro. 2010. *The State of Happiness: Can Public Policy Shape People's Wellbeing and Resilience?* London: Young Foundation.

Baker, S. and B. J. Brown. 2007. *Rethinking Universities: The Social Functions of Higher Education*. London and New York: Continuum International Publishers.

Barrett, D. and P. Hennessy. 2010. 'Mothers "betrayed" by Tories: Cameron was "untruthful" for promising us longer prison sentences, say victims' families'. *Sunday Telegraph*, 19 December.

Batt-Rawden, K. and G. Tellnes. 2011. 'How music may promote healthy behavior'. *Scandinavian Journal of Public Health* 39 (2): 113–20.

Baum, M. A. and P. B. K. Potter. 2008. 'The Relationships between Mass Media, Public Opinion, and Foreign Policy: Toward a Theoretical Synthesis'. *Annual Review of Political Science* 11: 39–65.

Bauman, Z. 1988. *Freedom*. Buckingham: Open University Press.

———. 1989. *Legislators and Interpreters*. Cambridge: Polity.

———. 1997. *Postmodernity and Its Discontents*. Cambridge: Polity.

———. 2000. *Liquid Modernity*. Cambridge: Polity.

———. 2002. 'Foreword: Individually, Together'. In *Individualization*, ed. U. Beck and E. Beck-Gernsheim. London: Sage Publications.

Baxter, K. and C. Glendinning. 2011. 'Making Choices About Support Services: Disabled Adults' and Older People's Use of Information'. *Health and Social Care in the Community* 19 (3): 272–79.

BBC. 2005. 'Carer jailed over sexual activity'. http://news.bbc.co.uk/1/hi/wales/north_east/4745431.stm (accessed 7 July 2011).

———. 2006. 'Mother allowed baby son's murder'. http://news.bbc.co.uk/1/hi/wales/south_west/6107138.stm (accessed 27 February 2011).

———. 2008. 'Teachers backing Baby P director'. http://news.bbc.co.uk/1/hi/england/london/7730817.stm (accessed 27 February 2011).

———. 2009. 'Baby death case worker reinstated'. http://news.bbc.co.uk/1/hi/wales/south_west/8270389.stm (accessed 27 February 2011).

———. 2010a. 'German girl band star charged in HIV case'. http://news.bbc.co.uk/1/hi/world/europe/8512933.stm (accessed 21 August 2010).

———. 2010b. 'Suspended sentence for German HIV singer Nadja Benaissa'. http://www.bbc.co.uk/news/world-europe-11097298 (accessed 19 February 2011).

———. 2010c. 'UK house prices: July-September 2010'. http://news.bbc.co.uk/1/shared/spl/hi/in_depth/uk_house_prices/html/houses.stm (accessed 6 January 2011).

———. 2010d. 'Paris Hilton sued over wearing "wrong hair extensions"'. http://www.bbc.co.uk/newsbeat/10951105 (accessed 19 February 2011).

———. 2011a. 'Half of Welsh women report mental health problems'. http://www.bbc.co.uk/news/uk-wales-12156198 (accessed 27 February 2011).

———. 2011b. 'MP Graham Allen calls for early years education'. http://www.bbc.co.uk/news/education-12216967 (accessed 26 February 2011).

————· 2011c. 'Narberth mother killing review finds agency "failings"'. http://www.bbc. co.uk/news/uk-wales-12149278 (accessed 8 December 2011).

Beck, U. 1992. *Risk Society: Towards a New Modernity*. London: Sage Publications.

Beck, U. and E. Beck-Gernsheim. 2002. *Individualization*. London: Sage Publications.

Beckett, K. and B. Western 2001. 'Governing Social Marginality: Welfare, Incarceration, and the Transformation of State Policy'. In *Mass Imprisonment in the United States*, ed. D. Garland, 35–50. London: Sage Publications.

Bellah, R. N., R. Madsen, W. M. Sullivan, A. Swidler and S. M. Tipton. 1985. *Habits of the Heart: Individualism and Commitment in American Life*. Berkeley: University of California Press.

Bellamy, R. 2008. *Citizenship: A Very Short Introduction*. Oxford: Oxford University Press.

Bender, A. and C. Ewashen. 2000. 'Group Work is Political Work: A Feminist Perspective of Interpersonal Group Psychotherapy'. *Issues in Mental Health Nursing* 21: 297–308.

Bennett, A. 2011. 'The post-subcultural turn: Some reflections 10 years on'. *Journal of Youth Studies* 14 (5): 493–506.

Berger, P. L. 1977. *Facing Up to Modernity: Excursions in Society, Politics and Religion*. New York: Basic Books.

Berk, L., K. T. Hallam, F. Colom, E. Vieta, M. Hasty, C. Macneil and M. Berk. 2010. 'Enhancing Medication Adherence in Patients with Bipolar Disorder'. *Human Psychopharmacology* 25: 1–16.

Bernstein, B. 2001. 'Symbolic Control: Issues of Empirical Description of Agencies and Agents'. *International Journal of Social Research Methodology* 4 (1): 21–33.

Berridge, V. 2009. 'Medicine, public health and the media in Britain from the nineteen-fifties to the nineteen-seventies'. *Historical Research* 82 (216): 360–73.

Besley, A. C. 2005. 'Jim Marshall: Foucault and Disciplining the Self'. *Educational Philosophy and Theory* 37 (3): 309–15.

Bevan, G. and C. Hood. 2006. 'Have Targets Improved Performance in the English NHS?' *British Medical Journal* 332: 419–22.

Beveridge, W., 1942. *Social Insurance and Allied Services*. New York: Macmillan.

Biggs, D., N. Hovey, P. J. Tyson and S. MacDonald. 2010. 'Employer and employment agency attitudes towards employing individuals with mental health needs'. *Journal of Mental Health* 19 (6): 509–16.

Bigo, D. 2002. 'Security and Immigration: Toward a Critique of the Governmentality of Unease'. *Alternatives* 27: 63–92.

Bjorklund, P. 2004. '"There but for the grace of god": Moral Responsibility and Mental Illness'. *Nursing Philosophy* 5: 188–200.

Blake, H. 2010. 'Man charged after hospital row over his mother's care: Solicitor is denied access to ward and then arrested'. *Daily Telegraph*, 24 August.

Blaxter, M. 1983. 'The Causes of Disease: Women Talking'. *Social Science and Medicine* 17: 5969.

Blaxter, M. and N. Britten. 1996. 'Lay Beliefs about Drugs and Medicines and the Implications for Pharmacy'. Manchester: Pharmacy Practice Research Resource Centre.

Bloxham, A. 2010. 'Call obese people fat says minister'. *Daily Telegraph*, 29 July.

Blumer, H. 1969. *Symbolic Interactionism: Perspective and Method*. Berkeley: University of California Press.

Bottero, W. 2010. 'Intersubjectivity and Bourdieusian approaches to "identity"'. *Cultural Sociology* 4 (1): 3–22.

Bourdieu, P. 1990. *The Logic of Practice*. Cambridge: Polity.

————· 1998. 'The essence of neoliberalism'. *Le Monde Diplomatique*, 8 December. http://mondediplo.com/1998/12/08bourdieu (accessed 1 August 2010).

————· 1999. *Acts of Resistance: Against the Tyranny of the Market*. New York: New Press.

Bourgois, P. 2000. 'Disciplining Addictions: The Bio-politics of Methadone and Heroin in the United States'. *Culture, Medicine and Psychiatry* 24: 165–95.

Bradley, Lord. 2009. *The Bradley Report: Lord Bradley's review of people with mental health problems or learning disabilities in the criminal justice system*. London: Department of Health.

Bradley, Q. 2008. 'Capturing the castle: tenant governance in social housing companies'. *Housing Studies* 23 (6): 879–897.

————· 2011. 'Trouble at the Top: The Construction of a Tenant Identity in the Governance of Social Housing Organizations'. *Housing, Theory and Society* 28 (1): 19–38.

Briscoe, C. 2006. *Ugly*. London: Hodder and Stoughton.

Britten, N. 2001. 'Prescribing and the Defence of Clinical Autonomy'. *Sociology of Health and Illness* 23 (4): 478–96.

Brodie, J. 2007. 'Reforming Social Justice in Neoliberal Times'. *Studies in Social Justice* 1: 93–107.

Brooks, R. and S. Goldstein. 2006. *The Power of Resilience: Achieving Balance, Confidence and Personal Strength in Your Life*. New York: McGraw-Hill.

Brown, B. and P. Crawford. 2007. 'Personality Disorder in UK Mental Health Care: Language, Legitimation and the Psychodynamics of Surveillance'. In *Hospital Communication*, ed. R. Iedema, 109–37. London: Palgrave Macmillan.

————· 2009. '"Post Antibiotic Apocalypse": Discourses of Mutation in Narratives of MRSA'. *Sociology of Health and Illness* 31 (4): 508–24.

Brown, P. 2008. 'Legitimacy Chasing its Own Tail: Theorising Clinical Governance Through a Critique of Instrumental Reason'. *Social Theory and Health* 6: 184–99.

Brown, P. and M. Calnan. 2009. 'The Risks of Managing Uncertainty: The Limitations of Governance and Choice, and the Potential for Trust'. *Social Policy and Society* 9 (1): 13–24.

Bunton, R. 1997. 'Popular Health, Advanced Liberalism and Good Housekeeping Magazine'. In *Foucault, Health and Medicine*, ed. A. Petersen and R. Bunton, 223–47. London: Routledge.

Bunton, R. and R. Burrows. 1995. 'Consumption and Health in the "Epidemiological" Clinic of Late Modern Medicine'. In *The Sociology of Health Promotion*, ed. R. Bunton, S. Nettleton and R. Burrows, 206–22. London: Routledge.

Burchell, G. 1996. 'Liberal Government and Techniques of the Self'. *Foucault and Political Reason: Liberalism, Neo-Liberalism, and Rationalities of Government*, ed. A. Barry, T. Osborne and N. Rose, 19–36. Chicago: University of Chicago Press.

Burrows, M. and S. Greenwell. 2007. 'The Other End of the Telescope: A Refocusing of Mental Health and Well Being for Service Users and Carers'. Report of All Wales Review of Mental Health Services.

Buttny, R. 2004. *Talking Problems: Studies on Discursive Construction*. Albany, NY: State University of New York Press.

Byrne, R. 2006. *The Secret*. New York: Simon & Schuster.

Cabinet Office. 1999. 'Modernising Government'. London: The Stationery Office.

————· 2010. 'The Coalition: Our Programme for Government: Freedom, Fairness Responsibility'. London: Cabinet Office.

————· 2011. 'Building a new culture of social responsibility'. London: Cabinet Office.

Callinicos, A. 1989. *Against Postmodernism: A Marxist Critique*. London: Polity.

Calnan, M. 1987. *Health and Illness: The Lay Perspective*. London: Tavistock.

Calnan, M. and R. Rowe. 2008. *Trust Matters in Healthcare*. Buckingham: Open University Press.

Campbell, A. 2011, *Diaries, vol. 2: Power and the People*. London: Hutchinson.

Campbell, P. 1996. 'The History of the User Movement in the United Kingdom'. In *Mental Health Matters*, ed. T. Heller, T. Reynolds and J. Gomm. Basingstoke: Palgrave Macmillan.

———. 2001. 'The Role of Users of Psychiatric Services and Service Development Influence Not Power'. *Psychiatric Bulletin* 25: 87–8.

Caplan, J. and J. Torpey. 2001. 'Introduction'. In *Documenting Individual Identity: The Development of State Practices in the Modern World*, ed. J. Caplan and J. Torpey. Princeton: Princeton University Press.

Capps, D. 1993. *The Depleted Self: Sin in a Narcissistic Age*. Minneapolis: Fortress.

Carey, M. 2009. 'Happy Shopper? The Problem with Service User and Carer Participation'. *British Journal of Social Work* 39: 179–88.

Carlen, P. and J. Tombs. 2006. 'Reconfigurations of Penality: The Ongoing Case of the Women's Imprisonment and Reintegration Industries'. *Theoretical Criminology* 10 (3): 337–60.

Carnegie, D. 1936. *How to Win Friends and Influence People*. New York: Simon & Schuster.

Carpenter, H. 1991. 'A victim of suburbia'. *Sunday Times*, 22 December.

Carr, H. 2010. 'Looking Again at Discipline and Gender: Theoretical Concerns and Possibilities In the Study of Anti-Social Behaviour Initiatives'. *Social Policy and Society* 9 (1): 77–87.

Carr, S. 2007. 'Participation, Power, Conflict and Change: Theorizing Dynamics of Service User Participation in the Social Care System of England and Wales'. *Critical Social Policy* 27 (2): 266–76.

Carter, P. 2010. 'I won't let my girls wait until they're 25 before they have a smear test'. *Mail on Sunday*, 8 August.

Carvel, J. 2006. 'NHS criticised over mental health patient's death under restraint'. *Guardian*, 24 October.

Chaney, D. 1994. *The Cultural Turn: Scene-Setting Essays on Contemporary Cultural History*. London: Routledge.

Chandiramani, R. 2010. 'The Shoesmith Interview: "I haven't been able to move on at all"'. *Children and Young People Now*. http://www.cypnow.co.uk/news/1045184/Shoesmith-Interview-I-havent-able-move-all/ (accessed 27 February 2011).

Channel 4. 2010. *The Fairy Jobmother*, series 1, episode 1, 13 July 2010. http://www.channel4.com/programmes/the-fairy-jobmother/episode-guide/series-1/episode-1. (accessed 6 December 2011).

Chavez, L. R., F. A. Hubbell, J. M. McMullin, R. G. Martinez and S. I. Mishra. 1995. 'Structure and Meaning in Models of Breast and Cervical Cancer Risk Factors: A Comparison of Perceptions Among Latinas, Anglo Women, and Physicians'. *Medical Anthropology Quarterly* 9 (1): 40–74.

Chomsky, N. 2011. *Profit Over People: Neoliberalism And Global Order*. New York: Seven Stories Press.

Christopher, J. C. and S. Hickinbottom. 2008. 'Positive Psychology, Ethnocentrism and the Disguised Ideology of Individualism'. *Theory and Psychology* 18 (5): 563–89.

Clark, R. 2006. *How to Label a Goat: The Silly Rules and Regulations That Are Strangling Britain*. London: Harriman House.

Clarke, J. 2004. 'Subjects of Doubt: In Search of the Unsettled and the Unfinished'. Paper presented at the CASCA Conference, Ontario, 5–9 May 2004.

————. 2005. 'New Labour's Citizens: Activated, Empowered, Responsibilized, Abandoned?' *Critical Social Policy* 25: 447–63.

————. 2010. 'Public Management or Managing the Public? The Frank Stacey Memorial Lecture 2009, presented at the Public Administration Committee Conference, University of Glamorgan, 8 September 2009'. *Public Policy and Administration* 25 (3): 1–7.

Clarke, J., J. Newman and L. Westmarland. 2007. 'The Antagonisms of Choice: New Labour and the Reform of Public Services'. *Social Policy and Society* 7 (2): 245–53.

Clough, P. T. 2004. 'Future Matters: Technoscience, Global Politics, and Cultural Criticism'. *Social Text* 22 (3): 1–23.

————. 2008. 'The Affective Turn: Political Economy, Biomedia and Bodies'. *Theory, Culture and Society* 25 (1): 1–22.

Cobb, N. 2006. 'Patronising the Mentally Disordered? Social Landlords and the Control of 'Anti-social Behaviour' Under the Disability Discrimination Act 1995'. *Legal Studies* 26 (2): 238–66.

Cochrane, D. 1989. 'Poverty, Probation and Empowerment'. *Probation Journal* 36 (4): 177–82.

Coleman, J. S. 1982. *The Asymmetric Society.* Syracuse, NY: Syracuse University Press.

Collins, M. 2010. 'From "sport for good" to "sport for sport's sake" – not a good move for sports development in England?" *International Journal of Sports Policy and Politics* 2 (3): 367–79.

Collins, P. 2008. 'The Continuing Horror Story of Spiegelgrund: Mental Health, Compassion, Awareness and Incarceration'. *Journal of Prisoners on Prisons* 17 (2): 6–15.

Condor, S. 2011. 'Towards a social psychology of citizenship?' *Journal of Community and Applied Social Psychology* 21: 293–301.

Condron, S. 2007. 'Attacks on nurses "cost £100m a year"'. *Daily Telegraph*, 26 February.

Conrad, P. 2007. *The Medicalization of Society: On the Transformation of Human Conditions into Treatable Disorders.* Baltimore: Johns Hopkins University Press.

Conway, M. A. 1990. *Autobiographical Memory: An Introduction.* Milton Keynes: Open University Press.

Covey, S. R. 1989. *The Seven Habits of Highly Effective People.* New York: Free Press.

Cowan, D. and A. Marsh. 2005. 'From Need to Choice, Welfarism to Advanced Liberalism? Problematics of Social Housing Allocation'. *Legal Studies* 25 (1): 22–48.

Cowan, D. and M. McDermont. 2006. *Regulating Social Housing: Governing Decline.* New York: Routledge-Cavendish.

Coward, R. 1989. *The Whole Truth: The Myth of Alternative Health.* London: Faber & Faber.

Cowden, S. and G. Singh. 2007. 'The "User": Friend, Foe or Fetish? A Critical Exploration of User Involvement in Health and Social Care'. *Critical Social Policy* 27 (5): 5–23.

Cox, R. S., B. C. Long, M. I. Jones and R. J. Handler. 2008. 'Sequestering of Suffering: Critical Discourse Analysis of Natural Disaster Media Coverage'. *Journal of Health Psychology* 13 (4): 469–80.

Coyne, A. 2002. 'Should patients who assault staff be prosecuted?' *Journal of Psychiatric and Mental Health Nursing* 9: 139–145.

Crawford, P. and B. Brown. 2008. 'Soft Authority: Ecologies of Infection Management in the Working Lives of Modern Matrons and Infection Control Staff'. *Sociology of Health and Illness* 30 (5): 756–71.

Cress, D. M. and D. A. Snow. 2000. 'The Outcomes of Homeless Mobilization: The Influence of Organization, Disruption, Political Mediation, and Framing'. *American Journal of Sociology* 105 (4): 1063–1104.

Crow, T. J. 2008. 'The emperors of the schizophrenia polygene have no clothes'. *Psychological Medicine* 38: 1681–5.

Cruikshank, B. 1996. 'Revolutions within: Self-government and self-esteem'. In *Foucault and Political Reason: Liberalism, Neo-Liberalism, and Rationalities of Government*, ed. A. Barry, T. Osborne and N. Rose. Chicago: University of Chicago Press.

———. 1999. *The Will to Empower: Democratic Citizens and Other Subjects*. Ithaca, NY: Cornell University Press.

Csikszentmihalyi, M. 1997. *Finding Flow: The Psychology of Engagement with Everyday Life*. New York: Basic Books.

———. 1999. 'If We're So Rich Why Aren't We Happy?' *American Psychologist* 54: 821–7.

Curtis, P. 2008. '"We have to take responsibility": Christine Gilbert tells Polly Curtis what Baby P means for Ofsted and social services'. *Guardian*, 6 December.

D'Ancona, M. 2010. 'We are seeing an audacious challenge to the orthodoxy; the manic row over child benefit has eclipsed the true radicalism of the Tory leader's strategy'. *Sunday Telegraph*, 10 October.

Daily Post. 2004. 'Mentally ill man has to spend day in car: No care for son whilst mother is in college'. *Daily Post*, 4 December.

Daily Telegraph. 2010a. 'Town hall litter fine for ex-mayor'. *Daily Telegraph*, 30 October.

———. 2010b. 'Labour has created 4,300 offences'. *Daily Telegraph*, 2 March.

Dalrymple, T. 2005. 'In the Asylum'. *City Journal*. http://www.city-journal.org/html/15_3_oh_to_be.html (accessed 19 February).

Das, V. 2004. 'The signature of the state: the paradox of illegibility'. *Anthropology in the margins of the state*, ed. V. Das and D. Poole, 225–52. Oxford: James Currey.

———. 2011. 'State, citizenship, and the urban poor'. *Citizenship Studies* 15 (3–4): 319–33.

Davies, N. 2004. 'Trapped in a cycle of self-harm and despair for want of a psychiatric bed'. *Guardian*, 7 December.

de Graaf, J., D. Wann and T. H. Naylor. 2001. *Affluenza: The All Consuming Epidemic*. New York: Berrett-Koehler Publishers.

Deacon, A. 2004. 'Justifying conditionality: The case of anti-social tenants'. *Housing Studies* 19 (6): 911–26.

Dean, C. E. 2011. 'Psychopharmacology: A House Divided'. *Progress in Neuro-Psychopharmacology & Biological Psychiatry* 35 (1): 1–10.

Dean, M. 1999. *Governmentality: Power and Rule in Modern Society*. London: Sage Publications.

———. 2002. 'Powers of Life and Death Beyond Governmentality'. *Cultural Value* 6: 119–38.

———. 2007. *Governing Societies: Political Perspectives on Domestic and International Rule*. Maidenhead: Open University Press.

Deary, I. J. and G. D. Batty. 2007. 'Cognitive Epidemiology'. *Journal of Epidemiology and Community Health* 61: 378–84.

Deary, I. J., C. R. Gale, M. C. W. Stewart, F. G. R. Fowkes, G. D. Murray, G. D. Batty and J. F. Price. 2009. 'Intelligence and persisting with medication for two years: Analysis in a randomised controlled trial'. *Intelligence* 37: 607–12.

Delgado, M. 2008. 'New job for boss axed in superbug row…advising the NHS'. *Mail on Sunday*, 27 January.

Department for Communities and Local Government. 2011. 'A new mandatory power of possession for anti-social behaviour'. London: Department for Communities and Local Government.

Department for Work and Pensions. 2006. 'A new deal for welfare: Empowering people to work'. London: HMSO.

———· 2008. 'No one written off: Reforming welfare to reward responsibility'. London: The Stationery Office.

———· 2010. 'Universal Credit: Welfare that works'. London: The Stationery Office.

Department of the Environment, Transport and the Regions (DETR) 2000. 'Quality and Choice: A Decent Home for All: The Housing Green Paper'. London: Department of the Environment, Transport and the Regions.

Department of Health. 1998. 'Modernising mental health services: Safe, sound and supportive'. London: Department of Health.

———· 1999. 'National service framework for mental health: Modern standards and service models'. London: Department of Health.

———· 2004. 'Choosing health: Making healthy choices easier'. London: Department of Health.

———· 2005. 'Independence, Wellbeing and Choice: Our Vision for the Future of Adult Care'. London: Department of Health.

———· 2008. 'Transforming social care'. London: Department of Health.

———· 2010. 'Equity and excellence: Liberating the NHS'. London: Department of Health.

Department of Health and Social Security. 1976. 'Prevention and health, everybody's business: A reassessment of public and personal health'. London: HMSO.

Derbyshire, D. 2010. 'Getting your recycling wrong will cost you more than shoplifting'. *Daily Mail*, 26 November.

Deutsch, N. L. and E. Theodorou. 2010. 'Aspiring, Consuming, Becoming: Youth Identity in a Culture of Consumption'. *Youth and Society* 42 (2): 229–54.

Dillane, J., M. Hill, J. Bannister and S. Scott. 2001. *Evaluation of the Dundee Families Project*. Edinburgh: Scottish Executive.

Djulbegovic, M., R.J. Beyth, M. N. Neuberger, T. L. Stoffs, J. Vieweg, B. Djulbegovic and P. Dahm. 2010. 'Screening for prostate cancer: Systematic review and meta-analysis of randomised controlled trials'. *British Medical Journal* 341: 4543–552.

Donnelly, L., M. Howie, B. Leach. 2010. 'Councils pay for prostitutes for the disabled'. *Daily Telegraph*. http://www.telegraph.co.uk/health/7945785/Councils-pay-for-prostitutes-for-the-disabled.html (accessed 7 December 2011).

Donovan, J. L. and D. R. Blake. 1992. 'Patient non-compliance: Deviance or reasoned decision-making?' *Social Science and Medicine* 34: 50713.

Donovan, N. and D. Halpern. 2002. 'Life Satisfaction: The state of knowledge and implications for government'. London: Prime Minister's Strategy Unit.

Dowling, S., Manthorpe, J. and S. Cowley. 2006. 'Person-centred planning in social care: A scoping review'. Kings College London, Social Care Workforce Research Unit. York: York Publishing Services Ltd.

Downes, D. 2007. 'Visions of Penal Control in the Netherlands'. In *Crime, Punishment, and Politics in Comparative Perspective: Crime and Justice, vol. 36*, ed. M. Tonry, 93–125. Chicago: University of Chicago Press.

Dreyfus, H. L. and P. Rabinow. 1982. *Michel Foucault: Beyond Structuralism and Hermeneutics*. Chicago: University of Chicago Press.

du Gay, P. 2000. 'Entrepreneurial Governance and Public Management: The Anti-Bureaucrats'. In *New Managerialism New Welfare?*, ed. J. Clarke, S. Gewirtz and E. McLaughlin. London: Sage Publications.

Duits, L. and P. V. R. Vis. 2009. 'Girls make sense: Girls, celebrities and identities'. *European Journal of Cultural Studies* 12 (1): 41–58.

Dwyer, P. 1998. 'Conditional citizens: Rights and responsibilities in the late 1990s'. *Critical Social Policy* 18 (57): 493–517.

———. 2004. *Understanding Social Citizenship.* Bristol: The Policy Press.

Dyer, R. 1991. '"A Star is Born" and the Construction of Authenticity'. In *Stardom: Industry of Desire*, ed. C. Gledhill, 132–40. London: Routledge.

Eaton, B. C. and M. Eswaran. 2009. 'Well-being and Affluence in the Presence of a Veblen Good'. *Economic Journal* 119: 1088–1104.

Eckert, J. 2011. 'Introduction: Subjects of citizenship'. *Citizenship Studies* 15 (3–4): 309–17.

Edernariam, A. 2009. 'In her first interview since being dismissed as head of Haringey's children's services over the Baby P case, Sharon Shoesmith tells her side of the story'. *Guardian*, 7 February.

Edgar, D. 2007. 'These medical moralisers might as well try banning sex'. *Guardian*, 7 June.

Ehrenreich, B. 2009. *Smile or Die: How Positive Thinking Fooled America and the World.* London: Granta Books.

Eli Lilly. 2009. *For Family and Friends.* http://www.zyprexa.com/sch/forfamilyandfriends.jsp (accessed 16 July 2009).

Elliott, R. and K. Wattanasuwan. 1998. 'Brands as symbolic resources for the construction of identity'. *International Journal of Advertising* 17: 131–44.

Ellis, C. 2009. *Revision: Autoethnographic Reflections on Life and Work.* Walnut Creek: Left Coast Press.

Elshtain, J. B. 1995. *Democracy on Trial.* New York: Basic Books.

Elstad, T. A. and A. H. Eide. 2009. 'User participation in community mental health services: Exploring the experiences of users and professionals'. *Scandinavian Journal of Caring Sciences* 23: 674–81.

Emerson, R. W. 1979. *Collected Works of Ralph Waldo Emerson, vol. 2.* Cambridge, MA: Harvard University Press.

Enstrom, J. E. and G. C. Kabat. 2003. 'Environmental Tobacco Smoke and Tobacco Related Mortality in a Prospective Study of Californians, 1960-98'. *British Medical Journal* 326: 1057–1067.

Erikson, E. H. 1959. *Identity and the Life Cycle.* New York: W. W. Norton & Company.

———. 1968. *Identity, Youth and Crisis.* New York: W. W. Norton & Company.

Evans, J., B. Davies and J. Wright (eds). 2004. *Body Knowledge and Control: Studies in the Sociology of Physical Education and Health.* London: Routledge.

Farrer, F. 2000. *A Quiet Revolution: Encouraging and Sharing Positive Values with Children.* London: Rider and Co.

Featherstone, M. 1991. *Consumer Culture and Postmodernism.* London: Sage Publications.

Ferlie, E., L. Ashburner, L. Fitzgerald and A. Pettigrew. 1996. *The New Public Management in Action.* Oxford: Oxford University Press.

Field, F. 2003. *Neighbours From Hell: The Politics of Behaviour.* London: Politico's.

Field, S. 2010. 'Don't take offence if we lecture you on how to stay alive and healthy'. *Observer*, 8 August.

Fincham, J. E. 2007. *Patient Compliance With Medications: Issues and Opportunities.* Binghamton, NY: Pharmaceutical Products Press.

Fine, M. and J. Ruglis. 2009. 'Circuits and Consequences of Dispossession: Racialized Realignment of the Public Sphere for US Youth'. *Transforming Anthropology* 17 (1): 20–33.

Fischer, M. A., M. R. Stedman and J. Lii. 2010. 'Primary medication non-adherence: Analysis of 195,930 electronic prescriptions'. *Journal of General Internal Medicine* 2 (4): 284–90.

Flegal, K. M. and B. I. Graubard. 2009. 'Estimates of excess deaths associated with body mass index and other anthropometric variables'. *American Journal of Clinical Nutrition* 89: 1213–19.

Flegal, K. M., B. I. Graubard, D. F. Williamson and M. H. Gail. 2005. 'Excess deaths associated with underweight, overweight, and obesity'. *Journal of the American Medical Association* 293: 1861–7.

Flint, J. F. 2003. 'Housing and ethopolitics: Constructing identities of active consumption and responsible community'. *Economy and Society* 32 (4): 611–29.

———. 2004. 'The Responsible Tenant: Housing Governance and the Politics of Behaviour'. *Housing Studies* 19 (6): 893–909.

Foss, A. and K. Trick. 1989. *St. Andrews Hospital Northampton: The First 150 Years.* Cambridge: Granta Editions.

Foucault, M. 1972. *The Archaeology of Knowledge and the Discourse on Language.* New York: Pantheon Press.

———. [1975] 1995. *Discipline and Punish: The Birth of the Prison.* New York: Vintage Books.

———. 1977. *Discipline and Punish: The Birth of the Prison.* New York: Vintage Books.

———. 1978. *Discipline and Punish: The Birth of the Prison.* New York: Pantheon.

———. 1980. *Power/knowledge.* Brighton: Harvester.

———. 1985. *The Use of Pleasure: The History of Sexuality, vol. 2.* New York: Vintage Books.

———. 1988. 'Technologies of the Self'. In *Technologies of the Self,* ed. L. H. Martin, H. Gutman and P. H. Hutton. Amherst: University of Massachusetts Press.

———. 1990. *The Care of the Self: The History of Sexuality, vol. 3.* London: Penguin.

———. 1991. 'Governmentality'. In *The Foucault Effect: Studies in Governmentality,* ed. G. Burchell, C. Gordon and P. Miller, 87–104. London: Harvester Wheatsheaf.

———. 1997. 'The Ethics of the Concern for Self as a Practice of Freedom'. In *Michel Foucault: Ethics, Subjectivity and Truth, the Essential Works of Michel Foucault 1954–1984, vol. 1,* ed. P. Rabinow. London: Penguin.

———. 2008. *The Birth of Biopolitics: Lectures at the Collège de France 1978–79,* trans. G. Burchell. Basingstoke: Palgrave Macmillan.

France, C. M., P. H. Lysaker and R. P. Robinson. 2007. 'The "Chemical Imbalance" Explanation for Depression: Origins, Lay Endorsement, and Clinical Implications'. *Professional Psychology: Research and Practice* 38 (4): 411–20.

Franco, E. L. 2009. 'Managing low grade and borderline cervical abnormalities: The dilemma of choosing between conservative and aggressive policies remains'. *British Medical Journal* 339: 305–6.

Freire, P. 1973. *Pedagogy of the Oppressed.* Harmondsworth: Penguin.

Frey, J. 2003. *A Million Little Pieces.* New York: Random House.

Fullagar S. 2009. 'Negotiating the neurochemical self: Anti-depressant consumption in women's recovery from depression'. *Health* 13 (4): 389–406.

Funiciello, T. 1993. *Tyranny of Kindness: Dismantling the Welfare System to End Poverty in America.* New York: Atlantic Monthly Press.

Furedi, F. 1997. *The Culture of Fear: Risk Taking and the Morality of Low Expectations.* London: Cassell.

———. 2002. 'Drug Control and the Ascendancy of Britain's Therapeutic Culture'. *In Drug Courts In Theory and in Practice,* ed. J. L. Nolan, 215–34. Hawthorne: Aldine De Grutyer.

————· 2003. *Therapy Culture: Cultivating Vulnerability in an Uncertain Age.* London: Routledge.

Gallie, W. B. 1956. 'Essentially Contested Concepts'. *Proceedings of the Aristotelian Society* 56: 167–98.

Gallivan, M. and G. Depledge. 2003, 'Trust, control and the role of interorganizational systems in electronic partnerships'. *Information Systems Journal* 13 (2): 159–90.

Garland, D. 1996. 'The Limits of the Sovereign State: Strategies of Crime Control in Contemporary Society'. *British Journal of Criminology* 36: 445–71.

————· 2001. *The Culture of Control: Crime and Social Order in Contemporary Society.* Oxford: Oxford University Press.

Garthwaite, K. 2011. '"The language of shirkers and scroungers?" Talking about illness disability and Coalition welfare reform'. *Disability and Society* 26 (3): 369–72.

Gellner, E. 1993. *The Psychoanalytic Movement: The Cunning of Unreason,* 2nd ed. London: Fontana Press.

George, U., B. Lee, S. McGrath and K. Moffatt. 2003. 'Exploring citizenship in contemporary community work practice'. *Journal of Community Practice* 11 (3): 71–86.

Gewirth, A. 1998. *Self-fulfilment.* Princeton: Princeton University Press.

Ghate, D. and M. Ramella. 2002. *Positive Parenting: The National Evaluation of the Youth Justice Board's Parenting Programme.* London: Youth Justice Board for England and Wales.

Giddens, A. 1990. *The Consequences of Modernity.* Cambridge: Polity.

————· 1991. *Modernity and Self-Identity: Self and Society in Late Modern Age.* Cambridge: Polity.

————· 1998. *The Third Way. The Renewal of Social Democracy.* Cambridge: Polity.

————· 2000. *The Third Way and its Critics.* Cambridge: Polity.

Gilmore, R. W. 2007. *Golden Gulag: Prisons, Surplus, Crisis, and Opposition in Globalizing California.* Berkeley: University of California Press.

Giroux, H. A. 2004. *The Terror of Neoliberalism: Authoritarianism and the Eclipse of Democracy.* New York: Paradigm.

————· 2009. *Youth in a Suspect Society: Democracy or Disposability?* New York: Palgrave Macmillan.

Glasby, J., J. Le Grand and S. Duffy. 2009. 'A healthy choice? Direct payments and healthcare in the English NHS'. *Policy and Politics* 37 (4): 481–97.

Glasby, J. and R. Littlechild. 2009. *Direct Payments and Personal Budgets: Putting Personalisation Into Practice,* 2nd ed. Bristol: The Policy Press.

Glass, N. and C. Moreton. 2001. 'An artist? I'm a brand name says Hirst'. *Independent,* 1 October.

Glaze, L. E. and T. Bonczar. 2006. 'Probation and Parole in the United States, 2005'. *Bureau of Justice Statistics Bulletin, Rev. January 18, 2007.* Washington, DC: US Department of Justice.

Glendinning, C. and P. Kemp (eds). 2006. *Cash and Care: Policy Challenges in the Welfare State.* Bristol: The Policy Press.

Gloucester Citizen. 2006. 'Please spray me with your CS gas'. *Gloucester Citizen,* 9 December.

Goldberg, D. 2005. 'The Disclosure Conundrum: How People with Psychiatric Disabilities Navigate Employment'. *Psychology, Public Policy, and Law* 11 (3): 463–500.

Goldenberg, J. L., C. Routledge and J. Arndt. 2009. 'Mammograms and the management of existential discomfort: Threats associated with the physicality of the body and neuroticism'. *Psychology and Health* 24 (5): 563–81.

Goldfinch, S. and J. Wallis. 2010. 'Two Myths of Convergence in Public Management Reform'. *Public Administration* 88 (4): 1099–1115.

Goleman, D. 1998. *Working with Emotional Intelligence*. London: Bloomsbury.

Goode, J., D. Greatbatch, A. O'Cathain, D. Luff, G. Hanlon and T. Strangleman. 2004. 'Risk and the Responsible Health Consumer: The Problematics of Entitlement among Callers to NHS Direct'. *Critical Social Policy* 24 (2): 210–32.

Gottschalk, M. 2009. 'The Long Reach of the Carceral State: The Politics of Crime, Mass Imprisonment, and Penal Reform in the United States and Abroad'. *Law & Social Inquiry* 34 (2): 439–72.

Gould, E. and E. Mitty. 2010. 'Medication Adherence is a Partnership, Medication Compliance is Not'. *Geriatric Nursing* 31 (4): 290–8.

Goulding, C., A. Shankar and M. Elliott. 2002. 'Working Weeks, Rave Weekends: Identity Fragmentation and the Emergence of New Communities'. *Consumption, Markets and Culture* 5 (4): 261–84.

Grant, E. 2010. 'Writing the reflexive self: An autoethnography of alcoholism and the impact of psychotherapy culture'. *Journal of Psychiatric and Mental Health Nursing* 17: 577–82.

Gray, R. 2006. 'Hospital "time waster" files used to flag up repeat A&E attenders'. *Scotland on Sunday*, 9 April.

Greco, M. 1993. 'Psychosomatic subjects and the "duty to be well"'. *Economy and Society* 22: 357–72.

Greer, S., S. Moorey, J. D. R. Baruch, M. Watson, B. M. Robertson, A. Mason, L. Rowden, M. G. Law and J. M. Bliss. 1992. 'Adjuvant psychological therapy for patients with cancer: A prospective randomised trial'. *British Medical Journal* 304: 675–80.

Grey, C. 1997. 'Management as a Technical Practice: Professionalization or Responsibilization?' *Systems Practice* 10 (6): 703–25.

Grice, A. 2010. 'Prime minister unveils happiness index'. *Independent*, 25 November.

Gronniger, J. T. 2005. 'A Semiparametric Analysis of the Body Mass Index's Relationship to Mortality'. *American Journal of Public Health* 96: 173–8.

Grotz, M., U. Hapk, T. Lampert and H. Baumeister. 2011. 'Health locus of control and health behaviour: Results from a nationally representative survey'. *Psychology, Health and Medicine* 16 (2): 129–40.

Grover, C. and L. Piggott. 2010. 'From Incapacity Benefit to Employment and Support Allowance: Social Sorting, Sickness and Impairment, and Social Security'. *Policy Studies* 31 (2): 265–82.

Gueguen, N. and M. Vion. 2009. 'The effect of a practitioner's touch on a patient's medication compliance'. *Psychology, Health and Medicine* 14 (6): 689–94.

Guignon, C. B. 2004. *On Being Authentic*. New York: Routledge.

Habermas, J. 1984. *The Theory of Communicative Action, vol. 1: Reason and the Rationalisation of Society*. Boston: Beacon Press.

———. 1987. *The Theory of Communicative Action, vol. 2: Lifeworld and System: A Critique of Functionalist Reason*. Cambridge: Polity.

Hall, C. 1997. *Social Work as Narrative: Storytelling and Persuasion in Professional Texts*. Aldershot: Ashgate.

Hallowell, N. 1998. 'You don't want to lose your ovaries because you think, "I might become a man"'. Women's perceptions of prophylactic surgery as a cancer risk management option'. *Psycho-Oncology*, 7: 263–75.

Halse, C. 2007. 'The Bio-citizen: Virtue Discourses, BMI and Responsible Citizenship, Paper Presented at the Bio-pedagogies Conference'. University of Wollongong, January.

Hamilton, C. and R. Denniss. 2005. *Affluenza: When Too Much is Never Enough*. London: Allen and Unwin.

Harcourt, B. E. 2010. 'Neoliberal Penality: A Brief Genealogy'. *Theoretical Criminology* 14 (1): 74–92.

Hardin, P. K. 2001. 'Theory and language: Locating agency between free will and discursive marionettes'. *Nursing Inquiry* 8: 11–8.

Harrison S. R. and C. Smith. 2003. 'Neo-bureaucracy and public management: The case of medicine in the National Health Service'. *Competition and Change* 7 (4): 243–54.

Harter, S. 1999. *The Construction of the Self: A Developmental Perspective*. New York: Guilford Press.

Harvey, A. 2010. 'Genetic risks and healthy choices: Creating citizen-consumers of genetic services through empowerment and facilitation'. *Sociology of Health and Illness* 32: 365–82.

Harvey, D. 2003. *A Brief History of Neoliberalism*. Oxford: Oxford University Press.

Hatton, C. and J. Waters. 2011. *National Personal Budget Survey June 2011*. Lancaster: Lancaster University/In Control.

Haworth, A. and T. Manzi. 1999. 'Managing the "Underclass": Interpreting the Moral Discourse of Housing Management'. *Urban Studies* 36 (1): 793–806.

Healthcare Commission. 2006. 'Health watchdog highlights gaps in community mental health care'. http://www.healthcarecommission.org.uk/newsandevents/pressreleases (accessed 21 November).

Heelas, P. 1996. 'On Things not being Worse, and the Ethic of Humanity'. In *Detraditionalization*, ed. P. Heelas, S. Lash and P. Morris. London: Blackwell.

Henry, P. 2006. 'Magnetic points for lifestyle shaping: The contribution of self-fulfillment, aspirations, and capabilities'. *Qualitative Market Research: An International Journal* 9 (2): 170–80.

Henwood, M. and R. Hudson. 2008. 'Personalisation: A New Model for Integration?' *Journal of Integrated Care* 16 (3): 8–16.

Her Majesty's Government. 2007. 'Putting People First: A shared vision and commitment to the transformation of Adult Social Care'. London: Her Majesty's Government.

Her Majesty's Inspector of Constabulary (HMIC). 2010a. 'Antisocial behaviour: Stop the rot'. London: Her Majesty's Inspector of Constabulary.

———. 2010b. 'Stop the Drift: A Focus Upon 21st Century Criminal Justice'. London: Her Majesty's Inspector of Constabulary.

Herbert, I. 2005. 'Judge condemns care system after being forced to send mentally ill woman to jail'. *Independent*, 5 July.

Herrnstein, R. J. and C. Murray. 1994. *The Bell Curve*. New York: Free Press.

Hill, F. J. 2003. 'Complementary and alternative medicine: the next generation of health promotion?' *Health Promotion International* 18 (3): 265–72.

Hill, N. 1937. *Think and Grow Rich*. New York: The Ralston Society.

Hilliard, L. T. 1954. 'Resettling Mental Defectives: Psychological and Social Aspects'. *British Medical Journal* 4875: 1372–4.

Hindess, B. 1996. *Discourses of Power: From Hobbes to Foucault*. Oxford: Blackwell.

Hinsliff, G. 2005. 'Therapy for those seeking sick notes'. *Observer*, 20 November.

Hirschorn, L. 1997. *Reworking Authority: Leading and Following in the Post-modern Organisation*. Cambridge, MA: MIT Press.

Hodgkinson, S. and N. Tilley. 2011. 'Tackling anti-social behaviour: Lessons from New Labour for the Coalition Government'. *Criminology and Criminal Justice* 11 (4): 283–305.

Holmqvist, M. 2009. 'Medicalization of unemployment: Individualizing social issues as personal problems in the Swedish welfare state'. *Work, Employment and Society* 23 (3): 405–21.

Home Office. 2003. 'Respect and Responsibility – Taking a Stand Against Anti-Social Behaviour'. London: HMSO.

hooks, b. 1999. *Remembered Rapture: The Writer at Work*. London: Women's Press.

Hooper, L., C. Bartlett, G. Davey-Smith and S. Ebrahim. 2002. 'Systematic review of long term effects of advice to reduce dietary salt in adults'. *British Medical Journal* 325 (7365): 628–37.

House of Lords. 2006. *Economic Affairs Committee Fifth Report*. http://www.publications. parliament.uk/pa/ld200506/ldselect/ldeconaf/183/18302.htm (accessed 11 August 2011).

Hunt, H. and G. Wickham. 1994. *Foucault and Law*. London: Pluto Press.

Hunter, I. 1996. 'Assembling the School'. In *Foucault and Political Reason*, ed. A. Barry, T. Osborne and N. Rose, 143–66. London: UCL Press.

Ilcan, S. 2009. 'Privatizing Responsibility: Public Sector Reform Under Neoliberal Government'. *Canadian Review of Sociology* 46 (3): 207–34.

Ilkan, S. and T. Basok. 2004. 'Community government: Voluntary agencies, social justice, and the responsibilization of citizens'. *Citizenship Studies* 8: 129–44.

Illouz, E. 2008. *Saving the Modern Soul: Therapy, Emotions, and the Culture of Self-Help*. Berkeley: University of California Press.

In Control. 2006. *How to be in control*. DVD. Wythall: In Control.

Individual Budgets Evaluation Network. 2008. *Evaluation of the Individual Budgets pilot programme: Final report*. York: Individual Budgets Evaluation Network.

Institute for Government. 2010. *MINDSPACE: Influencing behaviour through public policy*. London: Institute for Government.

Isaacs, D. 2006. 'Attention-deficit/hyperactivity disorder: Are we medicating for social disadvantage?' *Journal of Paediatrics and Child Health* 42: 544–7.

Jacobs, D. H. 1995. 'Psychiatric drugging: Forty years of pseudo-science, self-interest and indifference to harm'. *Journal of Mind and Behaviour* 16 (4): 421–70.

Jago, B. J. 2011. 'Shacking Up: An Autoethnographic Tale of Cohabitation'. *Qualitative Inquiry* 17 (2): 204–19.

James, A. N. 2008. 'A critical consideration of the cash for care agenda and its implications for social services in Wales'. *Journal of Adult Protection* 10 (3): 23–34.

James, O. 2007. *Affluenza: How to Be Successful and Stay Sane*. London: Vermillion.

Jerome, J. 2011. 'Putting People First: 3rd Year Progress'. London: Social Care Transformation.

Johnston, P. 2010. *Bad Laws: An Explosive Analysis of Britain's Petty Rules, Health and Safety Lunacies and Madcap Laws*. London: Constable.

Jones, G. 2010. 'Proof the old police ways will beat the scum ruling our streets'. *Daily Express*, 26 June.

Jones, M. B. 2008. *Love and Consequences: A Memoir of Hope and Survival*. New York: Riverhead Books.

Jones, R., Pykett, J. and M. Whitehead. 2011. 'The Geographies of Soft Paternalism in the UK: The Rise of the Avuncular State and Changing Behaviour after Neoliberalism'. *Geography Compass* 5 (1): 50–62.

Jones, S. 2005. *Antonio Gramsci*. Oxford: Routledge.

Jordan, B. and C. Jordan. 2000. *Social Work and the Third Way*. London: Sage Publications.

Jorgensen, K. J. and P. C. Gøtzsche. 2009. 'Overdiagnosis in publicly organised mammography screening programmes: Systematic review of incidence trends'. *British Medical Journal* 339: b2587.

Kabat, G, 2008 *Hyping the Health Risks: Environmental Hazards in Daily Life and the Science of Epidemiology*. New York: Columbia University Press.

Kampman, O. and K. Lehtinen.. 1990. 'Compliance in psychosis'. *Acta Psychiatrica Scandinavica* 100: 167–75.

Kao, Y. C. and Y. P. Liu. 2010. 'Compliance and schizophrenia: The predictive potential of insight into illness, symptoms, and side effects'. *Comprehensive Psychiatry* 51 (6): 557–65.

Kazukauskas, K. A. and C. S. Lam. 2009. 'Disability and Sexuality: Knowledge, Attitudes, and Level of Comfort Among Certified Rehabilitation Counselors'. *Rehabilitation Counseling Bulletin* 54 (1): 15–25.

Kemshall, H. 2002a. 'Effective practice in probation: An example of "advanced liberal responsibilisation"?' *Howard Journal* 41: 41–58.

————. 2002b. *Risk, Social Policy and Welfare*. Buckingham: Open University Press.

Kenny, C. 2011. *Getting Better*. New York: Basic Books.

Kessler, R. C., P. Berglund, O. Demler, R. Jin, K. R. Merikangas and E. E. Walters. 2005. 'Lifetime prevalence and age-of-onset distributions of DSM-IV disorders in the National Comorbidity Survey Replication'. *Archives of General Psychiatry* 62: 593–602.

Kim, E. 2011. 'Asexuality in disability narratives'. *Sexualities* 14 (4): 479–93.

Kim, S. S. 2009. 'Individualism and Collectivism: Implications for Women'. *Pastoral Psychology* 58: 563–78.

Kmietowicz, Z. 2011. 'Trust defers surgical referrals for patients to lose weight and stop smoking'. *British Medical Journal*, doi:10.1136/bmj.d4792.

Koch, J. L. A. 1891. *Die Psychopathischen Minderwertigkeiten*. Dorn: Ravensburg.

Kollewe, J. 2010. 'Property: Nation of homeowners becomes a land of perpetual tenants: With prolonged housing crisis, big money is now moving into "build-to-let"'. *Guardian*, 18 December.

Korsgaard, C. M. 1996. *The Sources of Normativity*. Cambridge: Cambridge University Press.

Krugman, P. 2004. *Peddling Prosperity*. New York: W. W. Norton & Company.

Lalonde, M. 1974. *A New Perspective on the Health of Canadians: A Working Document*. Ottawa: Government of Canada.

Laude, A. and D. Tabuteau. 2007. *De l'observance a la gouvernance de sa sante*. Paris: Presses Universitaires de France.

Layard, R. 2007. 'Happiness and the teaching of values'. *CentrePiece* 12 (1): 18–23.

Leichter, H. M. 2003. '"Evil Habits" and "Personal Choices": Assigning Responsibility fir Health in the 20th Century'. *Milbank Quarterly* 81 (4): 603–26.

Lemke, T. 2001. 'The birth of bio-politics: Michael Foucault's lecture at the College de France on neo-liberal governmentality'. *Economy and Society* 30 (2): 190–207.

Lester, H. and J. Q. Tritter. 2005. 'Listen to my madness: Understanding the experiences of people with serious mental illness'. *Sociology of Health and Illness* 27 (5): 649–69.

Lindsay, J. 2010. 'Healthy living guidelines and the disconnect with everyday life'. *Critical Public Health* 20 (4): 475–87.

Lingam, R. and J. Scott. 2002. 'Treatment non-adherence in affective disorders'. *Acta Psychiatrica Scandinavica* 105: 164–72.

Link, L. B., L. Robbins, C. A. Mancuso and M. E. Charlson. 2004. 'How do cancer patients who try to take control of their disease differ from those who do not?' *European Journal of Cancer Care* 13: 219–26.

Lippman, A. 1991. 'Prenatal genetic testing and screening: Constructing needs and reinforcing inequalities'. *American Journal of Law and Medicine* 17 (1–2): 15–50.

Loewenthal, D. 2002. 'The nature of psychotherapeutic knowledge: Psychotherapy and counselling in universities'. *European Journal of Psychotherapy and Counselling* 5(4): 331–46.

Lowenberg, J. S. 1989. *Caring and Responsibility: The Crossroads Between Holistic Practice and Traditional Medicine*. Philadelphia: University of Pennsylvania Press.

Lowenheim, O. 2007. 'The Responsibility to Responsibilize: Foreign Offices and the Issuing of Travel Warnings'. *International Political Sociology* 1: 203–21.

Lubinski, D. 2009. 'Cognitive epidemiology: With emphasis on untangling cognitive ability and socioeconomic status'. *Intelligence* 37: 625–33.

Lukes, S. 1973. *Individualism*. London: Macmillan.

Lury, C. 1996. *Consumer Culture*. Cambridge: Polity.

Lyon-Callo, V. 2004. *Inequality, Poverty, and Neoliberal Governance: Activist Ethnography in the Homeless Sheltering Industry*. Orchard Park: Broadview Press.

MacDonald, S. 2006. 'A Suicidal Woman, Roaming Pigs and a Noisy Trampolinist: Refining the ASBO's Definition of "Anti-Social Behaviour"'. *Modern Law Review* 69 (2): 183–213.

MacIntyre, A. 1981. *After Virtue*. South Bend: University of Notre Dame Press.

Maclean, C. 2006. 'I'm with the brand: Craig Maclean spends an exhausting few days on the road with Paris Hilton: Singer, jewellery designer, socialite, entrepreneur, heiress, handbag maker, actress, nightclub owner, perfumer...' *Independent*, 13 August.

MacPherson, C. B. 1962. *The Political Theory of Possessive Individualism*. Oxford: Oxford University Press.

Maffesoli, M. 1988. 'Jeux de Masques: Postmodern Tribalism'. *Design Issues* 4 (1–2): 141–51.

Manza, J. and C. Uggen. 2006. *Locked Out: Felon Disenfranchisement and American Democracy*. New York: Oxford University Press.

Marcuse, H. 1989. 'From Ontology to Technology: Fundamental Tendencies of Industrial Society'. In *Critical Theory and Society: A Reader*, ed. S. Bronner and D. Kellner, 119–29. London: Routledge.

Marmot, M. 2010. *Fair Society, Healthy Lives: The Marmot Review*. London: The Marmot Review.

Marshall, J. D. 1996. *Michel Foucault: Personal Autonomy and Education*. Dordrecht: Kluwer Academic Publishers.

Marshall, J. D. and D. Marshall. 1997. *Discipline and Punishment in New Zealand Education*. Palmerston North: Dunmore Press.

Marshall, T. H. 1963. *Class, Citizenship, and Social Development*. Chicago: University of Chicago Press.

Martin, E. 1994. *Flexible Bodies: Tracking Immunity in American Culture from the Days of Polio to the Age of AIDS*. Boston: Beacon Press.

Martin, L. H., H. Gutman and P. Hutton (eds). 1988. *Technologies of the Self: A Seminar with Michael Foucault*. Amherst: University of Massachusetts Press.

Maryon-Davies, A. 2009. 'Why we need more nannying'. BBC News. http://news.bbc. co.uk/1/hi/health/7866833.stm (accessed 3 August 2010).

Mathieu, A. 1993. 'The Medicalization of Homelessness and the Theatre of Repression'. *Medical Anthropological Quarterly* 7 (2): 170–84.

Maudsley, H. 1884. *Body and Will: Being an Essay Concerning Will in its Metaphysical, Physiological, and Pathological Aspects*. New York: D. Appleton & Company.

Maynard, D. W. 1988. 'Language, Interaction and Social Problems'. *Social Problems* 35 (4): 311–34.

McAdams, D. P. 1997. *The Stories We Live By: Personal Myths and the Making of the Self*. New York: William Morrow.

McCartney, J. 2010a. 'Let's make it worthwhile to go to work'. *Sunday Telegraph*, 1 August.

———· 2010b. 'All puffed up like windy Stuart Baggs'. *Sunday Telegraph*, 19 December.

McClean, S. 2005. '"The illness is part of the person": Discourses of blame, individual responsibility and individuation at a centre for spiritual healing in the North of England'. *Sociology of Health and Illness* 27 (5): 628–48.

McCourt, F. 1996. *Angela's Ashes*. New York: Scribner Publishing.

McDonald, C. and G. Marston. 2005. 'Workfare as welfare: Governing unemployment in the advanced liberal state'. *Critical Social Policy* 25: 374–401.

McGinnis, J. M., P. Williams-Russo and J. R. Knickman. 2002. 'The Case for More Active Policy Attention to Health Promotion'. *Health Affairs* 21 (2): 78–93.

McGivern, G., M. Fischer, E. Ferlie and M. Exworthy. 2009. *Statutory Regulation and the Future of Professional Practice in Psychotherapy and Counselling: Evidence from the Field*. London: King's College London Economic & Social Research Council.

McGrath, C., C. F. C. Jordens, K. Montgomery and I. H. Kerridge. 2006. '"Right" way to "do" illness? Thinking critically about positive thinking'. *Internal Medicine Journal* 36: 665–8.

McIntyre, Z. and K. McKee. 2008. 'Governance and Sustainability in Glasgow: Connecting Symbolic Capital and Housing Consumption to Regeneration'. *Area* 40 (4): 481–90.

McKee, K. 2011. 'Sceptical, Disorderly and Paradoxical Subjects: Problematizing the "Will to Empower" in Social Housing Governance'. *Housing, Theory and Society* 28 (1): 1–18.

McKee, K. and V. Cooper. 2008. 'The paradox of tenant empowerment: Regulatory and liberatory possibilities'. *Housing, Theory and Society* 25 (2): 132–46.

McLaughlin, K. 2010. 'Psychologization and the construction of the political subject as a vulnerable object'. *Annual Review of Critical Psychology* 8: 63–79.

McPherson, K. 2010. 'Should We Screen for Breast Cancer?' *British Medical Journal* 341: 233–5.

McVeigh, T. 2010. 'Big Society: Power to the people, Cameron style: Lukewarm reception for the Tory leader's vision of self-help active communities'. *Observer*, 25 July.

Mennicken, A. 2008. 'Connecting worlds: The translation of international auditing standards into post-Soviet audit practice'. *Accounting, Organizations and Society* 33: 384–414.

Miller, P. and N. Rose. 1994. 'On therapeutic authority: Psychoanalytic expertise under advanced liberalism'. *History of the Human Sciences* 7 (3): 29–64.

———· 2008. *Governing the Present: Administering Economic, Social and Personal Life*. Cambridge: Polity.

Miller, R. B. and G. J. Maier. 1987. 'Factors Affecting the Decision to Prosecute Mental Patients for Criminal Behavior'. *Hospital and Community Psychiatry* 38: 50–5.

Milligan, M. and A. Neufeldt. 2001. 'The Myth of Asexuality: A Survey of Social and Empirical Evidence'. *Sexuality and Disability* 19 (2): 91–109.

Ministry of Justice. 2010. *Breaking the Cycle: Effective Punishment, Rehabilitation and Sentencing of Offenders*. London: Ministry of Justice.

Mitchell, T., 1999. 'Society, economy and the state effect'. In *State/Culture: State Formation after the Cultural Turn*, ed. G. Steinmetz, 76–97. Ithaca, NY: Cornell University Press.

Molz, J. 2005. 'Getting a "Flexible Eye": Round-the-World Travel and Scales of Cosmopolitan Citizenship'. *Citizenship Studies* 9: 517–31.

Monteith, B. 2009. *The Bully State: The End of Tolerance*. London: The Free Society.

Moore, D. 2009. '"Workers", "clients" and the struggle over needs: Understanding encounters between service providers and injecting drug users in an Australian city'. *Social Science and Medicine* 68: 1161–8.

Moore, M. 2009. 'Balls was reckless in Baby P affair says Shoesmith'. *Daily Telegraph*, 7 February.

Moorey, S. and S. Greer. 1989. *Psychological Therapy for Patients with Cancer*. Oxford: Heinemann Medical Books.

Morris, S. 2005. 'ASBO bars suicidal woman from rivers'. *Guardian*, 26 February.

Morrison, R. 2010. 'Election is about more than marking paper with a cross: Politics is in need of a revolution in trust and creativity which will open up a new chapter in democracy'. *Western Mail*, 15 April.

Morrow, N., O. Hargie, H. Donnelly and C. Woodman. 1993. '"Why do you ask?" A study of questioning behaviour in community pharmacist-client consultations'. *International Journal of Pharmacy Practice* 251: 90–4.

Mosher, C., G. Hooks and P. B. Wood. 2007. 'Don't Build It Here: The Hype Versus the Reality of Prisons and Local Employment'. In *Prison Profiteers: Who Makes Money from Mass Incarceration*, ed. T. Herivel and P. Wright, 90–7. New York: New Press.

NHS. 2004. *The New Community Pharmacy Framework*. London: The NHS Confederation.

———. 2005. *The National Health Service Act 1977: The Pharmaceutical Services (Advanced and Enhanced Services) (England) Directions 2005*. London: The Stationery Office.

———. 2009. *The NHS Constitution: The NHS belongs to us all*. London: National Health Service.

———. 2011. 'NHS Choices: Top 10 stress-busters'. http://www.nhs.uk/Livewell/Stressmanagement/Pages/Stressbusters.aspx (accessed 7 January 2011).

Nelson-Jones, R. 1979. 'Goals for counselling, psychotherapy and psychological education: Responsibility as an integrating concept'. *British Journal of Guidance and Counselling* 7 (2): 153–68.

Nettleton, S. and R. Bunton. 1995. 'Sociological Critiques of Health Promotion'. In *The Sociology of Health Promotion*, ed. R. Bunton, S. Nettleton and R. Burrows, 41–58. London: Routledge.

Newburn, T. 2007. 'Tough on crime: Penal policy in England and Wales'. In *Crime, Punishment, and Politics in Comparative Perspective, Crime and Justice, vol. 36*, ed. M. Tonry, 425–70. Chicago: University of Chicago Press.

Newnes, C. and N. Radcliffe. 2005. *Making and Breaking Children's Lives*. Ross-on-Wye: PCCS Books.

Niewhoner, J. 2011. 'Epigenetics: Embedded bodies and the molecularisation of biography and milieu'. *BioSocieties* 6: 279–98.

Nixon, J., C. Hunter, S. Parr, S. Whittle, S. Myers and D. Sanderson. 2006. 'Interim evaluation of rehabilitation projects for families at risk of losing their home as a result of anti-social behaviour'. London: Office of the Deputy Prime Minister.

Nolan, J. L. 1998. *The Therapeutic State*. New York: New York University Press.

Norcross, J. C., P. M. Krebs and J. O. Prochaska. 2011. 'Stages of change'. *Journal of Clinical Psychology* 67 (2): 143–54.

Norris, P. and B. Rowsell. 2003. 'Interactional issues in the provision of counselling to pharmacy customers'. *International Journal of Pharmacy Practice* 11: 135–42.

Novas, C. and N. Rose. 2000. 'Genetic risk and the birth of the somatic individual'. *Economy and Society* 29 (4): 485–513.

O'Donohoe, S. 1994. 'Advertising Uses and Gratifications'. *European Journal of Marketing* 28 (8–9): 52–75.

O'Grady, S. 2011. 'Bankruptcies down, but worries persist for 2011'. *Independent*, 5 February.

O'Mahony, C., N. Steedman, M. Yong, E. R. Anderson, V. Finnegan and L. Price. 2009. 'Let's not screen women under 25 throughout the UK'. *British Medical Journal* 339: b3426.

O'Malley, P. 1996. 'Risk and Responsibility'. In *Foucault and Political Reason: Liberalism, Neo-Liberalism and Rationalities of Government*, ed. A. Barry, T. Osborne and N. Rose, 189–207. London: UCL Press.

————. 2004. *Risk, Uncertainty and Government*. London: Routledge-Cavendish.

————. 2010. 'Resilient subjects: Uncertainty, warfare and liberalism'. *Economy and Society* 39 (4): 488–509.

O'Neill, B. 2010. 'A message to the illiberal nudge industry: Push off'. Spiked Online. http://www.spiked-online.com/index.php/site/article/9840/ (accessed 1 November).

O'Neill, O. 2002. *A Question of Trust*. Cambridge: Cambridge University Press.

Office for National Statistics. 2010. *Annual Survey of Hours and Earnings (ASHE) 2010*. London: Office of National Statistics. http://www.statistics.gov.uk/downloads/theme_labour/ashe-2010/2010-all-employees.pdf (accessed 6 January 2011).

Office of Public Service Reform. 2002. *Reforming our Public Services*. London: OPSR.

Olney, J. 1980. 'Autobiography and the Cultural Movement: A Thematic, Historical and Bibliographical Introduction'. In *Autobiography: Essays Theoretical and Critical*. Princeton: Princeton University Press.

Olson, E. 2008. 'The origins of European citizenship in the first two decades of European integration'. *Journal of European Public Policy* 15: 40–57.

Olstead, R. 2002. 'Contesting the text: Canadian media depictions of the conflation of mental illness and criminality'. *Sociology of Health and Illness* 24 (5): 621–43.

Ong, A. 1998. *Flexible Citizenship: the Cultural Logics of Transnationality*. Durham, NC: Duke University Press.

O'Toole, C. J. and J. K. Bregante. 1992. 'Disabled women: The myth of the asexual female'. In *Sex Equity and Sexuality in Education*, ed. S. S. Klein, 73–301. Albany, NY: SUNY Press.

Overholser, J. 2005. 'Contemporary Psychotherapy: Promoting personal responsibility for therapeutic change'. *Journal of Contemporary Psychotherapy* 35 (4): 369–76.

Page, B. I. 1996. 'The Mass Media as Political Actors'. *Political Science and Politics* 29 (1): 20–4.

Palazoolo, J. and J. P. Olie. 2004. *Observance Medicamenteuse et Psychiatrie*. Paris: Elsevier.

Parr, S. 2009. 'Confronting the reality of anti-social behaviour'. *Theoretical Criminology* 13: 363–81.

Parsons, E. and P. Atkinson. 1992. 'Lay constructions of genetic risk'. *Sociology of Health and Illness* 14: 437–55.

Pattillo-McCoy, M. 1999. *Black Picket Fences: Privilege and Peril among the Black Middle Class*. Chicago: University of Chicago Press.

Pauley, N. 2009. 'Jade death a massive life-saver: More women get cancer test'. *Daily Star*, 23 October.

Pawson, H. and R. Smith. 2009. 'Second generation stock transfers in Britain: Impacts on social housing governance and organisational culture'. *European Journal of Housing Policy* 9 (4): 411–33.

Peck, J. and A. Tickell. 2002. 'Neoliberalizing space'. In *Spaces of Neoliberalism: Urban Restructuring in North America and Western Europe*, ed. N. Brenner and N. Theodore, 34–57. Oxford: Blackwell.

Peet, R. 2007. *Geography of Power: Making Global Economic Policy*. London: Zed Books.

Pelzer, D. 1995. *A Child Called 'It': One Child's Courage to Survive*. New York: Health Communications Inc.

Perkins, R. and M. Rinaldi. 2002. 'Unemployment rates among patients with long-term mental health problems: A decade of rising unemployment'. *Psychiatric Bulletin* 26 (8): 295–8.

Perls, F., R. Hefferline and P. Goodman. 1951. *Gestalt Therapy: Excitement and Growth in the Human Personality*. New York: Julian Press.

Perron, A., C. Fluet and D. Holmes. 2005. 'Agents of care and agents of the state: Bio-power and nursing practice'. *Journal of Advanced Nursing* 50 (5): 536–44.

Perron, A., T. Rudge and D. Holmes. 2010. 'Citizen minds, citizen bodies: The citizenship experience and the government of mentally ill persons'. *Nursing Philosophy* 11: 100–11.

Peters, M. 2001. 'Education, Enterprise Culture and the Entrepreneurial Self: A Foucauldian Perspective'. *Journal of Educational Enquiry* 2 (2): 58–71.

Peters, T. 1987. *Thriving on Chaos: Handbook for a Management Revolution*. New York: Knopf.

_____. 1997. *Tom Peters' Career Survival Guide*. Boston: Houghton Mifflin.

Petersen, A. 1997. 'Risk, Governance and the New Public Health'. In *Foucault, Health and Medicine*, ed. A. Petersen and R. Bunton, 188–206. London: Routledge.

Petersen, A., M. Davies, S. Fraser and J. Lindsay. 2010. 'Healthy living and citizenship: An overview'. *Critical Public Health* 20 (4): 391–400.

Petersen, M. 2008. *Our Daily Meds: How the Pharmaceutical Companies Transformed Themselves into Slick Marketing Machines and Hooked the Nation on Prescription Drugs*. New York: Farrar, Straus and Giroux.

Philo, G. 1996. 'The media and public belief'. In *Media and Mental Distress*, ed. G. Philo. New York: Addison Wesley Longman.

Pilcher, J. 2011. 'No logo? Children's consumption of fashion'. *Childhood* 18 (1): 128–41.

Piche, J. and P. Larsen. 2010. 'The moving targets of penal abolitionism: ICOPA, Past, Present and Future'. *Contemporary Justice Review* 13 (4): 391–410.

Pitts-Taylor, V. 2010. 'The plastic brain: Neoliberalism and the neuronal self'. *Health* 14 (6): 635–52.

Piven, F. F. and R. A. Cloward. [1971] 1993. *Regulating the Poor: The Functions of Public Welfare*. New York: Vintage Books.

Platform 51. 2011. 'Women like me: Supporting wellbeing in girls and women'. London: Platform 51.

Porter, H. and A. Blair. 2006. 'Focus: Freedom and the law: Britain's liberties: The great debate'. *Observer*, 23 April.

Posner, R. A. 1985. 'An Economic Theory of the Criminal Law'. *Columbia Law Review* 85 (6): 1193–231.

Potter, J. 2000. 'Post-Cognitive Psychology'. *Theory and Psychology* 10: 31–7.

Power, M. 1997. *The Audit Society: Rituals of Verification*. Oxford: Oxford University Press.

Pratt, J. 2005a. *Penal Populism*. New York: Routledge.

_____. 2005b. 'Introduction'. In *The New Punitiveness: Trends, Theories, Perspectives*, ed. J. Pratt, D. Brown, M. Brown, S. Hallsworth and W. Morrison, xi–xxvi. London: Willan.

Prescott, J. and H. Davies. 2008. *Prezza, My Story: Pulling No Punches*. London: Headline.

Prichard, J. C. 1837. *A Treatise on Insanity and Other Disorders Affecting the Mind*. Philadelphia: Haswell, Barrington, and Haswell.

Prochaska, J. O. and C. C. DiClemente. 1983. 'Stages and processes of self-change of smoking: Toward an integrative model of change'. *Journal of Consulting and Clinical Psychology* 51: 390–5

Prochaska, J. O., C. C. DiClemente and J. C. Norcross. 1992. 'In search of how people change: Applications to addictive behavior'. *American Psychologist* 47: 1102–14.

Prochaska, J. O. and W. F. Velicer. 1997. 'The transtheoretical model of health behavior change'. *American Journal of Health Promotion* 12: 38–48.

Public Administration Select Committee (House of Commons). 2003. 'On Target? Government By Measurement'. London: The Stationery Office.

Purkiss, J. and D. Royston-Lee. 2009. *Brand You: Turn Your Unique Talents into a Winning Formula*. London: Artesian Publishers Ltd.

Pykett, D. 2007. 'Making citizens governable? The Crick Report as governmental technology'. *Journal of Education Policy* 22 (3): 301–19.

Pykett, J., R. Jones,, M. Whitehead, M. Huxley, K. Strauss, N. Gill, K. McGeevor, L. Thompson and J. Newman. 2011. 'Interventions in the political geography of "libertarian paternalism"'. *Political Geography* 30: 301–10.

Pykett, J., M. Seward and A. Schaefer. 2010. 'Framing the Good Citizen'. *British Journal of Politics and International Relations* 12: 523–38.

Rabiee, P. and N. Moran. 2006. 'Interviews with early individual budget holders'. York: Social Policy Research Unit, University of York.

Rabinow, P. and N. Rose. 2006. 'Biopower Today'. *Biosocieties* 1 (2): 195–217.

Radley, A. 1994. *Making Sense of Illness: The Social Psychology of Health and Disease*. London: Sage Publications.

Radway, J. A. 1984. *Reading the Romance: Women, Patriarchy and Popular Literature*. Chapel Hill: University of North Carolina Press.

Rakowski, W., J. P. Fulton and J. P. Feldman. 1993. 'Women's decision making about mammography: A replication of the relationship between stages of adoption and decisional balance'. *Health Psychology* 12: 209–14.

Rambo, C. 2007. 'Handing IRB an unloaded gun'. *Qualitative Inquiry* 13: 353–67.

Ramesh, R. 2011. 'Minister warns of cuts' impact on child carers'. *Guardian*, 4 October.

Ramesh, R. and P. Wintour. 2010. 'Anger over two-year tenancies and applicant curbs in housing shakeup: Plan "like deliberate attack on the poor" says Shelter: Leading Lib Dem labels reform "irrelevant fantasy"'. *Guardian*, 23 November.

Ramsay, P. 2008. 'The Theory of Vulnerable Autonomy and the Legitimacy of the Civil Preventative Order'. LSE Law, Society and Economy Working Papers. http://www.lse.ac.uk/collections/law/wps/WPS2008-01_Ramsay.pdf (accessed 28 December 2010).

———. 2009. 'The Theory of Vulnerable Autonomy and the Legitimacy of the Civil Preventative Order'. In *Regulating Deviance; Redirection of Criminalisation and the Futures of Criminal Law*, ed. B. McSherry, A. Norrie and S. Bronitt, 109–40. Oxford: Hart.

Randeria, S. 2007. 'The State of Globalization: Legal Plurality, Overlapping Sovereignties and Ambiguous Alliances Between Civil Society and the Cunning State in India'. *Theory, Culture and Society* 24 (1): 1–33.

Rantala, K. and T. Lehtonen. 2001. 'Dancing on the tightrope: Everyday aesthetics in the practice of shopping, gym experience and art making'. *European Journal of Cultural Studies* 4 (1): 63–83.

Reach, G. 2007. *Pourquoi se soigne-t-on?: Enquete sur la rationalite morale de l'observance*. Paris: Editions Le Bord de l'Eau.

Reece, H. 2000. 'Divorcing responsibly'. *Feminist Legal Studies* 8: 65–91.

Reiman, J. 2004. *The Rich Get Richer and the Poor Get Prison: Ideology, Class, and Criminal Justice*. Toronto: Allyn & Bacon.

Reivich, K. and A. Shatte. 2002. *The Resilience Factor: 7 Keys to Finding Your Inner Strength and Overcoming Life's Hurdles*. Chicago: Broadway Books.

Reynolds, G. P. and S. L. Kirk. 2010. 'Metabolic side effects of antipsychotic drug treatment – pharmacological mechanisms'. *Pharmacology and Therapeutics* 125: 169–79.

Richardson, F. C. 1989. 'Freedom and commitment in modern psychotherapy'. *Journal of Integrative & Eclectic Psychotherapy* 8: 303–19.

Richardson, L. 2000. 'Writing: A method of inquiry'. In *Handbook of Qualitative Research*, ed. N. K. Denzin and Y. S. Lincoln, 923–48. Thousand Oaks: Sage Publications.

Rizq, R. 2011. 'IAPT, anxiety and envy: A psychoanalytic view of NHS primary care mental health services today'. *British Journal of Psychotherapy* 27 (1): 37–55.

Roberts, C. 2006. '"What can I do to help myself?" Somatic individuality and contemporary hormonal bodies'. *Science Studies* 19 (2): 54–76.

Roberts, R. D., M. Zeidner and G. Matthews. 2001. 'Does emotional intelligence meet traditional standards for an intelligence? Some new data and conclusions'. *Emotion* 1: 196–231.

Ronai, C. 1995. 'Multiple reflections of child sex abuse: An argument for a layered account'. *Journal of Contemporary Ethnography* 23: 395–426.

Rose, H. 1994. *Love, Power and Knowledge: Towards a Feminist Transformation of the Sciences*. Cambridge: Polity.

Rose, N. 1990. *Governing the Soul: The Shaping of the Private Self*. London: Routledge.

———. 1993. 'Government, authority and expertise in advanced liberalism'. *Economy and Society* 22: 283–99.

———. 1996. *Inventing our Selves*. Cambridge: Cambridge University Press.

———. 1999. *Powers of Freedom: Reframing Political Thought*. Cambridge: Cambridge University Press.

———. 1999. *Governing the Soul: The Shaping of the Private Self*. Cambridge: Cambridge University Press.

———. 2000. 'The Biology of Culpability: Pathological Identity and Crime Control in a Biological Culture'. *Theoretical Criminology* 4 (1): 5–34.

———. 2001. 'Community, Citizenship and the Third Way'. In *Citizenship and Cultural Policy*, ed. D. Merydyth and J. Minson. London: Sage Publications.

———. 2007. *The Politics of Life Itself: Biomedicine, Power, and Subjectivity in the Twenty-First Century*. Princeton: Princeton University Press.

———. 2010. '"Screen and intervene": Governing risky brains'. *History of the Human Sciences* 23 (1): 79–105.

Rose, N. and P. Miller. 2010. 'Political Power beyond the State: Problematics of Government'. *British Journal of Sociology* 61 (s1): 271–303.

Rose, N. and C. Novas. 2004. 'Biological citizenship'. In *Global Assemblages: Technology, Politics, and Ethics as Anthropological Problems*, ed. A. Ong and S. J. Collier, 439–63. Oxford: Blackwell Publishing.

Rose, N. and T. Osborne. 2000. 'Governing cities, governing citizens'. In *Democracy, Citizenship and the Global City*, ed. E. Isin, 95–109. London: Routledge.

Rosenhan, D. L. 1973. 'On Being Sane in Insane Places'. *Science* 79: 250–8.

Rothstein, H. 2006. 'The institutional origins of risk: A new agenda for risk research'. *Health, Risk and Society* 8 (3): 215–21.

Roxburgh, R. 2011. 'Incapacity Benefit/Employment and Support Allowance migration pilots'. *Journal of Poverty and Social Justice* 19 (2): 181–3.

Salter, C. 2010. 'Compliance and concordance during domiciliary medication review involving pharmacists and older people'. *Sociology of Health and Illness* 32 (1): 21–36.

Samele, C., I. Seymour, B. Morris, A. Cohen E. Emerson. 2006. *Equal Treatment: Closing the Gap – Part 1 of the DRC's Formal Investigation Report*. London: Sainsbury Centre for Mental Health.

Sarup, M. 1993. *An Introductory Guide to Post-structuralism and Postmodernism*, 2nd ed. London: Harvester Wheatsheaf.

———. 1996. *Identity, Culture and the Postmodern World*. Edinburgh: Edinburgh University Press.

Sasieni, P., A. Castanon and J. Cuzick. 2009. 'Effectiveness of cervical screening with age: Population based case-control study of prospectively recorded data'. *British Medical Journal* 339: 328–34.

Sassoon, S. 1928. *Memoirs of a Fox-Hunting Man*. London: Faber & Faber.

———. 1930. *Memoirs of an Infantry Officer*. London: Faber & Faber.

Schafer, R. 1976. *A New Language for Psychoanalysis*. New Haven: Yale University Press.

Scheibe, K. E. 1986. 'Self-narrative and Adventure'. In *Narrative Psychology: The Storied Nature of Human Conduct*, ed. T. R. Sarbin, 129–151. New York: Praeger.

Schmidtz, D. and R. E. Goodin. 1998. *Social Welfare and Individual Responsibility*. Cambridge: Cambridge University Press.

Shotter, J. 1993. 'Psychology and citizenship: Identity and belonging'. In *Citizenship and Social Theory*, ed. B. Turner. London: Sage Publications.

Schou, I., Ø. Ekeberg and C. M. Ruland. 2005. 'The mediating role of appraisal and coping in the relationship between optimism – pessimism and quality of life'. *Psycho-oncology* 14: 718–27.

Schroevers, M. J., V. Kraaij and N. Garnefski. 2010. 'Cancer patients' experience of positive and negative changes due to the illness: Relationships with psychological well-being, coping, and goal reengagement'. *Psycho-oncology* 20: 165–72.

Schubert, S., S. Hansen, K. Dyer and M. Rapley. 2009. '"ADHD patient" or "illicit drug user"? Managing medico-moral membership categories in drug dependence services'. *Discourse and Society* 20 (4): 499–516.

Scourfield, P. 2005. 'Implementing the Community Care (Direct Payments) Act: Will the Supply of Personal Assistants Meet the Demand and at what Price?' *Journal of Social Policy* 34 (3): 1–20.

———. 2007. 'Social Care and the Modern Citizen: Client, Consumer, Service User, Manager and Entrepreneur'. *British Journal of Social Work* 37: 107–22.

Scull, A. T. 1984. *Decarceration: Community Treatment and the Deviant – A Radical View*, 2nd ed. Piscataway: Rutgers University Press.

Seeman, M. V. 2010. 'Schizophrenia: Women Bear a Disproportionate Toll of Antipsychotic Side Effects'. *Journal of the American Psychiatric Nurses Association* 16: (1): 21–9.

Seldon, A. 2010. *Trust: How We Lost It and How to Get it Back*, 2nd ed. London: Biteback.

Sellgren, K. 2011. 'MP Graham Allen calls for early years intervention'. http://www.bbc.co.uk/news/education-12216967 (accessed 2 February 2011).

Sender, K. 2006. 'Queens for a Day: Queer Eye for the Straight Guy and the Neoliberal Project'. *Critical Studies in Media Communication* 2 (23): 131–51.

Sennett, R. 1980. *Authority*. New York: Alfred A. Knopf.

———. 1998. *The Corrosion of Character: The Personal Consequences of Work in the New Capitalism*. New York: W. W. Norton & Company.

_____. 2008. *The Craftsman*. London: Allen Lane.

Shakespeare, T., K. Gillespie-Sells and D. Davies. 1996. *The Sexual Politics of Disability: Untold Desires*. London: Cassell.

Sharpe, D. 2010. 'Such absurdly draconian rules do nobody any favours'. *Independent*, 17 August.

Shepherd, J. 2010. 'Council illegally spied on family in "school cheating" case'. *Guardian*, 3 August.

Shugart, H. A. 2010. 'Consuming Citizen: Neoliberating the Obese Body'. *Communication, Culture and Critique* 3: 105–26.

Shute, S. 2004. 'The Sexual Offences Act 2003 (4): New Civil Preventative Orders Sexual Offences Prevention Orders; Foreign Travel Orders; Risk of Sexual Harm Orders'. *Criminal Law Review* 6: 417–40.

Sidakis, D. 2009. 'Private Military Companies and State Sovereignty: Regulating Transnational Flows of Violence and Capital'. In *Rules of Law and Laws of Ruling: On the Governance of Law*, ed. F. von Benda-Beckmann, K. von Benda-Beckmann and J. Eckert, 61–82. Farnham and Burlington: Ashgate.

Siebert, A. 2005. *The Resiliency Advantage: Master Change, Thrive Under Pressure, and Bounce Back From Setbacks*. Portland: Practical Psychology Press.

Simon, J. 2007. *Governing Through Crime: How the War on Crime Transformed American Democracy and Created a Culture of Fear*. Oxford: Oxford University Press.

Sims, P. 2010. 'Councils pay for disabled to visit prostitutes and lap-dancing clubs from £520mtaxpayerfund'. DailyMail.http://www.dailymail.co.uk/news/article-1303273/Councils-pay-disabled-visit-prostitutes-lap-dancing-clubs.html#comments (accessed 7 December 2011).

Skoglund, P., D. Isacson and K. I. Kjellgren. 2003. 'Analgesic medication – communication at pharmacies'. *Patient Education and Counseling* 51: 155–61.

Slack, J. 2010. 'To calm fears over 24 hour drinking labour vowed to bring in alcohol disorder zones: So in four years how many have been created? Not one.' *Daily Mail*, 18 February.

Slater, D. 1997. *Consumer Culture and Modernity*. Cambridge: Polity.

Smith, A. 2010. 'Mum says her son begged for help before his suicide'. *Camarthen Journal*, 18 August.

Smith, J. 2010. 'The woman in the dock can be the victim too'. *Independent*, 21 August. http://www.independent.co.uk/opinion/commentators/joan-smith/joan-smith-the-woman-in-the-dock-can-be-the-victim-too-2058877.html (accessed 21 August 2010).

Som, C. 2005. 'Nothing seems to have changed, nothing seems to be changing and perhaps nothing will change in the NHS: Doctors' response to clinical governance'. *International Journal of Public Sector Management* 18: 463–77.

Squire, C. 2010. 'Being naturalised, being left behind: The HIV citizen in the era of treatment possibility'. *Critical Public Health* 20 (4): 401–27.

St. Pierre, E. 2000. 'The Call for Intelligibility in Postmodern Educational Research'. *Educational Researcher* 29 (5): 25–8.

Stacey, J. 1997. *Teratologies: A Cultural Study of Cancer*. London: Routledge.

Stainton Rogers, W. 1991. *Explaining Health and Illness: An Exploration of Diversity*. Hemel Hempstead: Harvester Wheatsheaf.

Stanton, J. and P. Randall. 2011. 'Doctors accessing mental-health services: An exploratory study'. *British Medical Journal Open*, doi:10.1136/bmjopen-2010-000017.

Strauss, J. L. and S. J. Johnson. 2006. 'Role of treatment alliance in the clinical management of bipolar disorder, stronger alliances prospectively predict fewer manic symptoms'. *Psychiatry Research* 145: 215–23.

Sun. 2009. '178,000 women can't all be wrong; Jade's legacy as government blanks cancer plea, why?' *Sun*, 26 June.

Sylvester, R. and A. Thompson. 2010. 'It's loopy to think that locking everyone up will solve crime: Saturday interview'. *Times*, 11 December.

Szasz, T. S. 1974. *The Myth of Mental Illness*. New York: Harper & Row.

———. 1984. *The Therapeutic State: Psychiatry in the Mirror of Current Events*. New York: Prometheus Books.

Taylor, C. 1985. *Philosophical Papers, vol. 2. Philosophy and the Human Sciences*. New York: Cambridge University Press.

———. 1988. 'The Moral Topography of the Self'. In *Hermeneutics and Psychological Theory: Interpretive Perspectives On Personality, Psychotherapy and Psychopathology*, ed. S. B. Messer, L. A. Sass and R. L. Woolfolk, 298–320. New Brunswick: Rutgers University Press.

———. 1989. *Sources of the Self: The Making of the Modern Identity*. Cambridge, MA: Harvard University Press.

Taylor, S. E. 1983. 'Adjustment to Threatening Events: Theory of Cognitive Adaptation'. *American Psychologist* 58: 1161–73.

Taylor-Gooby, P. 2005. *Attitudes to Social Justice*. London: Institute for Public Policy Research.

———. 2008. *Reframing Social Citizenship*. Oxford: Oxford University Press.

Tejeda, S., B. Thompson, G. D. Coronado and D. P. Martin. 2009. 'Barriers and facilitators related to mammography use among lower educated Mexican women in the USA'. *Social Science and Medicine* 68: 832–9.

Thakkar, P. and R. Kini. 2009. 'Staff Attitudes on Reporting Physical Violence Perpetrated by Patients'. The Sixth National Conference on Research in Medium Secure Units, 29 January 2009. London: Kings College, Institute of Psychiatry.

Thaler, R. and C. Sunstein. 2008. *Nudge: Improving Decisions About Health, Wealth, and Happiness*. Cambridge: Yale University Press.

Thapar-Björkert, S. and K. J. Morgan. 2010. '"But Sometimes I Think…They Put Themselves in the Situation": Exploring Blame and Responsibility in Interpersonal Violence'. *Violence Against Women* 16 (1): 32–59.

Thompson, J. B. 1995. *The Media and Modernity: A Social Theory of the Media*. Cambridge: Polity.

———. 1996. 'Tradition and Self in a Mediated World'. In *Detraditionalisation*, ed. P. Heelas, S. Lash and P. Morris. London: Blackwell.

Thornicroft, G. 2006. *Shunned: Discrimination against people with mental illness*. Oxford: Oxford University Press.

Titscher, S., M. Meyer, R. Wodak and E. Vetter. 2000. *Methods of Text and Discourse Analysis*. London: Sage Publications.

Tocqueville, A. de. [1835] 1969. *Democracy in America*. New York: Anchor Books.

Tolich, M. 2009. 'A Critique of Current Practice: Ten Foundational Guidelines for Autoethnographers'. *Qualitative Health Research* 20 (12): 1599–1610.

TOMBOLA Group. 2009. 'Cytological surveillance compared with immediate referral for colposcopy in management of women with low grade cervical abnormalities: Multicentre randomised controlled trial'. *British Medical Journal* 339: b2546.

Tone, A. 2009. *The Age of Anxiety: A History of America's Turbulent Affair with Tranquilizers*. New York: Basic Books.

Toynbee, P. 2010. 'A red carpet of opportunity awaits shell-shocked Labour: Cameron will be doomed by his cuts and Clegg by his betrayal. Miliband can now win over voters as the honest politician'. *Guardian*, 14 December.

Travis, A. 2010. 'Thousands spied on by councils but few are prosecuted: 8,500 covert operations in two years, study finds vast majority uncover nothing, watchdog says'. *Guardian*, 24 May.

Triandis, H. C. 1995. *Individualism and Collectivism*. Boulder: Westview Press.

Tribunals Service. 2009. *Decision in the First Tier Tribunal (Health, Education and Social Care) Between Eleni Cordingley and the Care Council for Wales*. Cardiff: Tribunals Service (Care Standards).

Trostle, J. A. 1988. 'Medical Compliance as an Ideology'. *Social Science and Medicine* 27: 1299–1308.

Tyler, R. 2011. 'Employers have duty to nudge staff into good health'. *Daily Telegraph*, 8 February.

Ubel, P. A. and G. Loewenstein. 1997. 'The role of decision analysis in informed consent: Choosing between intuition and systematicity'. *Social Science and Medicine* 44 (5): 647–56.

Ungar, S. and D. Bray. 2005. 'Silencing science: partisanship and the career of a publication disputing the dangers of second hand smoke'. *Public Understanding of Science* 14: 5–23.

Ungerson, C. and S. Yeandle (eds). 2007. *Cash for Care in Developed Welfare States*. Basingstoke: Palgrave Macmillan.

Urquhart, F. 2009. 'Asbo man "breaks law" by laughing'. *Scotland on Sunday*, 6 December.

US Preventive Services Task Force. 2009. 'Screening for Breast Cancer: U.S. Preventive Services Task Force Recommendation Statement'. *Annals of Internal Medicine* 151: 716–26.

Valverde, M. 1999. *Diseases of the Will*. Cambridge: Cambridge University Press.

Verhoeff, B. 2010. 'Drawing borders of mental disorders: An interview with David Kupfer'. *BioSocieties* 5: 467–75.

Villadsen K. 2008. 'Freedom as self-transgression: Transformations in the "governmentality" of social work'. *European Journal of Social Work* 11 (2): 93–104.

Vrecko, S. 2010. 'Neuroscience, power and culture: An introduction'. *History of the Human Sciences* 23 (1): 1–10.

Wacquant, L. 2002. 'The Curious Eclipse of Prison Ethnography in the Age of Mass Incarceration'. *Ethnography* 3 (4): 371–97.

_____· 2007. *Deadly Symbiosis: Race and the Rise of Neoliberal Penality*. Cambridge: Polity.

_____· 2008. 'Ordering Insecurity: Social Polarization and the Punitive Upsurge'. *Radical Philosophy Review* 11 (1): 9–27.

_____· 2009. *Prisons of Poverty: Expanded Edition*. Minneapolis: University of Minnesota Press.

Wahl, O. 1995. *Media Madness: Public Images of Mental Health*. New Brunswick: Rutgers University Press.

Waldby, C. and M. Cooper. 2008. 'The Biopolitics of Reproduction'. *Australian Feminist Studies* 23 (55): 57–73.

Waldron, S. 2010. 'Measuring Subjective Wellbeing in the UK'. London: Office of National Statistics.

Wales Audit Office. 2005. 'Adult mental health services in Wales: A baseline review of service provision'. Cardiff: Wales Audit Office.

_____· 2008. 'Joint Review of Gwynedd Council Social Services'. Cardiff: Care and Social Services Inspectorate Wales.

Walker, J. 2005. 'When the mentally ill commit crimes'. *Independent*, 29 September.

Walker, K. 2006. 'Smokers and the obese may get a second-class NHS'. *Daily Mail*, 27 December.

Walker, M. 1996. 'It's Superwoman: She has kept a Park Avenue apartment for seven years using it only to change clothes'. *Guardian*, 15 April.

Walker, R. M., G. A. Brewer, G. A. Boyne and C. N. Avellaneda. 2011. 'Market Orientation and Public Service Performance: New Public Management Gone Mad'. *Public Administration Review* 71 (5): 707–17.

Wallston, B. S. and K. A. Wallston. 1978. 'Locus of Control and Health: A Review of the Literature'. *Health Education Monographs* 6: 107–17.

Warhurst, C. and D. Nickson. 2001. *Looking Good, Sounding Right: Style Counselling and the Aesthetics of the New Economy*. London: The Industrial Society.

Washington, D. M. and D. G. Beecher. 2011. 'Music as Social Medicine: Two Perspectives on the West Eastern Divan Orchestra'. *New Directions for Youth Development* 125: 127–40.

Wattles, W. D. 1910. *The Science of Getting Rich*. New York: Elizabeth Towne.

Weaver, V. M. and A. E. Lerman. 2010. 'Political Consequences of the Carceral State'. *American Political Science Review* 104 (4): 817–33.

Webb, S. A. 2006. *Social Work in a Risk Society: Social and Political Perspectives*. Basingstoke: Palgrave Macmillan.

Weber, M. 1978. *Weber: Selections in Translation*. Cambridge: Cambridge University Press.

Western Mail. 2010. 'Singing is a wonderful way of promoting wellbeing. It lifts the mood, removes stress and makes people feel better'. *Western Mail*, 6 December.

White, M. 2005. 'The liberal character of ethological governance'. *Economy and Society* 34 (3): 474–94.

Whitehead, T. 2010a. 'Courts allow more serial criminals to stay on the street; 56,000 hardened offenders escaped jail terms'. *Daily Telegraph*, 29 December.

———. 2010b. 'Justice is being strangled with red tape'. *Daily Telegraph*, 3 November.

Wighton, K. 2010. 'We Only Had Cancer Test Thanks to Jade… She Saved Our Lives; Jade's Legacy One Year On: The Women She Saved'. *Sun*, 18 March.

Wilkinson, S. and C. Kitzinger. 2000. 'Thinking Differently About Thinking Positive: A Discursive Approach to Cancer Patients' Talk'. *Social Science and Medicine* 50: 797–811.

Willetts, D. 2010. 'Happiness is not… an attack on free markets; don't dismiss the link between wealth and wellbeing. They are driven by the same things'. *Times*, 26 November.

Williams, S. J. and M. Calnan. 1996. *Modern Medicine: Lay Perspectives and Experiences*. London: UCL Press.

Williams, N. 2009. 'Staff "relief" at exposed failings'. *South Wales Evening Post*, 2 April.

Williams, Z. 2009. 'Can't fix it till you feel it: The offer of therapy for the unemployed ignores the inconvenient fact that life isn't always fair'. *Guardian*, 11 March.

Williamson, J. 1990. 'What Washington Means By Policy Reform'. In *Latin American Adjustment: How Much Has Happened?* ed. J. Williamson, 7–20. Washington, DC: Institute for International Economics.

Willse, C. 2010. 'Neo-liberal biopolitics and the invention of chronic homelessness'. *Economy and Society* 39 (2): 155–84.

Wilson, D. 2006. 'Seduced by the politics of penal populism'. *Independent*, 16 August.

Wilson, J. Q. and G. Kelling. 1982. 'Broken Windows: The Police and Neighbourhood Safety'. *Atlantic Monthly* 249 (3): 29–38.

Winnett, R. 2011. 'Cameron: Our crisis of confidence'. *Daily Telegraph*, 25 July.

Wintour, P. 2010. 'Cameron tells nation: Pull together and we'll survive hard times ahead: PM attempts to revive "Big Society" idea: Child benefits cut is fair, he tells Tory conference'. *Guardian*, 7 October.

Wittchen, H.U., F. Jacobi, J. Rehm, A. Gustavsson, M. Svensson, B. Jönsson, J. Olesen, C. Allgulander, J. Alonso, C. Faravelli, F. Fratiglioni, P. Jennum, R. Lieb, A. Maercker, J. van Os, M. Preisig, L. Salvador-Carulla, R. Simon and H.C. Steinhausen. 2011. 'The size and burden of mental disorders and other disorders of the brain in Europe 2010'. *European Neuropsychopharmacology* 21: 655–79.

World Health Organization. 2003. *Adherence to Long-Term Therapies: Evidence for Action.* Geneva: World Health Organization.

Wright, J. K. 2009. 'Autoethnography and Therapy: Writing on the Move'. *Qualitative Inquiry* 15 (4): 623–40.

Yalom, I. D. 1980. *Existential Psychotherapy*. New York: Basic Books.

Yau, Y. 2011. 'On the anti-social behaviour control in Hong Kong's public housing'. *Housing Studies* 26 (5): 701–22.

Yeandle, S. and C. Ungerson. 2007. 'Conceptualizing Cash for Care: The Origins of Contemporary Debates'. In *Cash for Care in Developed Welfare States*, ed. C. Ungerson and S. Yeandle. Basingstoke: Palgrave Macmillan.

Yeoman, F. 2009. 'Singer with most popular German band faces jail for "infecting man with HIV"'. *Times*, 14 April. http://entertainment.timesonline.co.uk/tol/arts_and_entertainment/entertainment_news/article6092258.ece (accessed 8 August 2010).

Young, J. 1999. *The Exclusive Society: Social Exclusion, Crime and Difference in Late Modernity.* London: Sage Publications.

Zedner, L. 2006. 'Policing Before and After the Police'. *British Journal of Criminology* 46: 78–96.

INDEX

Lightning Source UK Ltd.
Milton Keynes UK
UKOW040720310812

198314UK00002B/7/P